**Paula Bartimeus** is a professional nutritionist and a regular writer for health magazines.

# Eating with the
# SEASONS

*How to Achieve Health and Vitality
by Eating in Harmony with Nature*

PAULA BARTIMEUS

E L E M E N T

Shaftesbury, Dorset • Boston, Massachusetts
Melbourne, Victoria

First published in Great Britain in 1998 by
Element Books Limited
Shaftesbury, Dorset SP7 8BP

Published in the USA in 1998 by
Element Books, Inc.
160 North Washington Street, Boston, MA 02114

Published in Australia in 1998 by
Element Books and distributed
by Penguin Books Australia Ltd
487 Maroondah Highway, Ringwood,
Victoria 3134

Lines taken from 'The Scene Changes', 'The Wind in the
Wheatfield', 'Music in the Mist' and 'Walking on a Winter's
Day' in Through the Year with Patience Strong (Random House,
London, 1996) reproduced by kind permission of Patience
Strong and Rupert Crew Literary Agents.

Design by Roger Lightfoot
Plate photographs by Iain Bagwell
Typeset by Footnote Graphics, Warminster, England
Printed and bound in Great Britain by
Creative Print & Design, Wales

British Library Cataloguing in Publication
data available

Library of Congess Cataloging in Publication
data available

ISBN 1 86204 201 2

This book is dedicated to my spiritual teacher Sri Chinmoy, who has helped me see that today's inspiring dreams are tomorrow's aspiring realities. I offer him my utmost love and deepest gratitude.

# Acknowledgements

I would like to offer my thanks first to my parents, Alma and Len, for their continuing support in whatever I choose to do. Also to my husband, Ben, for his encouragement and patience. To Barbara Wrenn, Principal of the College of Natural Nutrition, for all the amazing knowledge she shares; to Wendy Mandy, for her insight and understanding; and to Kleo Fanthorpe, for her many healing gifts. And last but not least, to Charlotte, my dear little guinea pig, who accompanied me through my long hours of writing this book.

# Contents

# List of Figures

# Introduction

According to the ancient Chinese the secret of good health was to live in harmony with nature. This was achieved by observing the natural flow of things and existing off the land. They adapted their lives from season to season and ate, worked and slept around this unending cycle.

It is unfortunate that in our modern society we have moved away from this simple existence. We no longer abide by the laws of the universe and we live in a fragmented world, cut off from its elements. If we desire to be happy on all levels, we must find our way back to this natural way of being.

In this book, I have set out to show that the age-old principles revered by the Chinese (and other cultures) still apply today.

As a nutritionist, I believe that the most fundamental link we have with nature is through our diet. By eating the food that grows around us from season to season, we can maintain our connection with the earth and receive the best nourishment to support and balance us.

For example, in the spring, when greens are abundant, we can use them to cleanse and purify our system, washing away the stagnant winter load. When summer arrives we are provided with the juiciest of fruits to keep us cool and hydrated. And as we move into the colder seasons, once again the autumn harvest and hearty winter roots will see us through.

Following such a system encourages us to go beyond single nutritional ideas and concepts. It rejects the lack of compromise and rigidity of specific practices and instead integrates all of them into one.

Having dabbled in several food philosophies over the years, I have come to the conclusion that extracting the most apt from the many is the right way to go. Regimes such as macrobiotics, the raw revolution, food combining and fasting all have much to offer; it's just knowing when to apply and possibly modify each one. For instance, eating a mainly raw food diet may be fine in the summer, but in the winter – not so kind. Here a more cooked, macrobiotic regime is preferable. Of course individual needs and personal preferences must also be taken into account.

*Eating with the Seasons* also takes a compassionate stand in its outlook, by supporting a vegetarian/vegan ideal. For reasons of disease prevention, ethics and spirituality, this, I feel, is the only way forward.

Within the following pages you'll find plenty of practical information on how to adjust your diet according to geographic location and time of year. Although the emphasis is based around temperate localities, it can easily be adapted to anyone, living anywhere. In general those who reside in polar or tropical regions, where the climate is relatively devoid of change, eat a similar diet all year round. The rest of us, who live in less extreme zones, experience the seasons more fully and need to tailor our diet appropriately.

Before we begin to make this transition we must first become acquainted with the basics of nutrition and how it affects us. This is covered in the first three chapters. Although this sidetracks away from the main theme of the book, please be patient – there's much in store. Like a tree that cannot bear fruit unless it's properly fed and watered, the foundations for health must first be laid before we can bloom.

Once we have attempted to make positive alterations in our dietary plan, we can move on and discover the rewards of eating with the seasons.

# CHAPTER 1

# Healthy Foundations

It's now generally accepted that the food we eat has a direct link to our state of health. If we choose to consume fresh, good-quality produce, then our quality of life will also be good. If we fill our bellies with processed, nutrientless junk, inevitably our health will suffer.

Having worked as a nutritionist for the last 14 years, I have witnessed the power of the plate time and time again, both by observing the improvements in others and through my own personal experience. These first few years employed as a health adviser were tremendously rewarding. As the doors opened to a new understanding, I began to realize the great impact our meals have on our well-being – both physically and mentally. I've seen people, young and old, from all walks of life, with all kinds of problems, help themselves back to good health, just by making a few sensible dietary changes. I must hasten to add that the healing process was often enhanced by the use of natural medicines, but I doubt the effects would have been so permanent if these individuals had not pursued a holistic approach. Of course, there were always a few who refused, point blank, to make any changes in what they ate – even if they were in obvious pain or discomfort. They were searching for that magic formula they'd heard of or read about and were unable to commit themselves to their own self-healing. Needless to say, they didn't return and I never saw them again.

The sooner we begin to take responsibility for our own health and nourish our bodies appropriately, the closer we'll be to leading a disease-free life. If we desire abundant energy, young-looking skin, a clear mind and a chance to live life to the full, then we must look to the very basics to claim our birthright. There are other factors that influence our health besides food that also need to be considered, but as we turn to a more positive way of being, these everyday essentials will naturally follow.

The nourishment we receive from our food, like all other life on this planet, is what our bodies are ultimately made of. Protein, fat and carbohydrate, together with vitamins and minerals and a supply of fresh water, all play a vital role in building, working and sustaining our system. If any one of these is lacking or in excess, the human machinery will eventually start to play up. With this in mind we can begin to understand the importance of nutrition and the effect it has on our inner mechanics.

Some years ago, when food was in short supply and nutrition was inadequate, deficiency diseases were prevalent. Scurvy, rickets and beriberi are common examples and have been the cause of many deaths. Yet although these afflictions have for the most part been wiped from the Western world, we are faced with a great deal of malnutrition. It's not due to a lack of food but rather to the dietary choices people are making.

For many of us, eating properly has gone out the window. We're so busy with our hectic, round-the-clock lives that even having one wholesome meal a day is off the agenda. Instead a variety of refined, so-called convenience foods is on the menu, marketed especially for the fast pace of life. These denatured food fixes have been robbed of the vital nutrients and fibres that keep us in good condition and in their place we now find sugar, salt and fat – three of the most notorious contributors to ill health. These items not only provide poor nutritional value, but actually cause a nutrient debt, as our bodies scramble to cope with the task of metabolizing them.

Excess protein from meat and the over-consumption of dairy foods have also created a sick picture. Tea and coffee have become popular addictions and even our fresh fruit and vegetables are subjected to the manhandling of commercial progress.

So we may not have to worry about the development of serious deficiency diseases any more, but instead we have other nutritional-related epidemics on our hands. A host of relatively new disorders, both chronic and acute, are now featured widely in our 'civilized' environment and the occurrence is steadily rising.

Heart disease, cancer, diabetes, asthma, arthritis, gallstones and infertility are just a few of the many problems modern-day living has brought with it. Some minor ailments are so common we even accept them as being normal. We blame the cold weather for our colds and the pollen for our hay fever. We even use the mild excuse of age for our aches and pains.

The truth of the matter is that we wouldn't have to put up with any of these maladies if we decided to take the right action. If the knowledge we have of nutrition today was applied to its full potential, most if not all twentieth-century diseases could be eventually eradicated. What we have to do is stop making excuses and start making changes. Then, and only then, will we have hope for a more healthful future.

## THE RIGHT DIET

Contrary to what many of us were brought up to believe, the basis of a healthy diet is far from the traditionally accepted meat and two veg. And while the marketing ploys aimed at us from infancy to adulthood may have rubbed off, they're slowly being replaced with other, less conventional schools of nutritional thought. Alongside the lobby for burgers, chips and cola is a growing industry for natural wholefoods and the 'new age' sustenance is catching on fast.

Although ideas on the ideal dietary practice can at times be conflicting, there are certain principles that largely seem to be agreed upon. Wholegrains, vegetables, beans and pulses, fruit, seeds and nuts have all been given the green flag, whilst the odd free-range egg and small amounts of goat's milk products are often also recommended. Whether to include animal-based produce in the diet or not will of course depend on individual wishes and requirements. But abstaining from them at least three days a week has been shown to aid the cleansing process of the body, preventing the accumulation of mucus and stagnant waste.

Another important advantage of consuming a diet based on plant foods is its ability to help stabilize the acid/alkaline balance of the blood. Food can be classified as either acid-forming or alkaline-forming, depending on the residue it leaves behind after being metabolized.[1] To maintain the ideal balance a greater proportion of alkaline-forming foods needs to be eaten.

Unfortunately, the average Western diet tends to lean more to the high acid intake, so it's not surprising that acidic conditions are so common.

Because the blood has to maintain a stable equilibrium, when we over-consume acidic foods the body tries to rectify the problem before a life-threatening situation occurs. It does this by ushering excess acidic substances out of the blood into surrounding tissues and joints, thus causing symptoms such as muscle aches, rheumatism and gout. Vital minerals (taken from the blood and bones) that act as buffers are also used up in a bid to neutralize the imbalance, leading to mineral deficiencies and illness.

Whilst over-alkalinity is comparatively rare, those following a totally raw food diet may be susceptible. But unlike acidic afflictions, problems associated with too much alkaline can easily be corrected, just by adding some grain to the diet.

Figure 1 shows how different foods compare. Entrants under the very acid-forming category should be as far as possible avoided. Mildly acid-forming foods are best eaten in a 40 per cent ratio, with alkaline-forming produce making up the remainder of the diet. Please bear in mind that this proportion may differ according to season and climate, people living in warmer areas possibly requiring a larger proportion of alkaline-forming foods.

Although I'm a great believer in 'everything in moderation', there are certain foods that are best avoided, for numerous reasons which will be covered later. Most of these are highly acid-forming and are the harbingers of ill health. Red meat, chemicalized salt,

*Figure 1, The acid- or alkaline-forming potential of different foods*

| | Alkaline-forming | Mildly acid-forming | Very acid-forming |
|---|---|---|---|
| Grains | amaranth<br>buckwheat<br>quinoa<br>sprouted grains<br>millet | barley<br>brown rice<br>corn<br>oats<br>rye<br>spelt<br>wheat<br>bread | refined grains |
| Legumes | sprouted beans/<br>    pulses | beans<br>lentils<br>peas<br>tofu<br>tempeh | peanuts |
| Vegetables[2] | All vegetables,<br>    including<br>    potatoes and<br>    seaweed, are<br>    alkaline-forming | | |
| Fruit | Almost all fruit,<br>    including citrus<br>    and dried fruit,<br>    is alkaline-<br>    forming | avocado | cranberries<br>rhubarb<br>sour plums<br>prunes<br>unripe fruit |
| Nuts | almonds<br>Brazil nuts | cashews<br>hazelnuts<br>pecans<br>macadamia nuts<br>walnuts | |
| Seeds | linseeds<br>sprouted seeds | hemp<br>pumpkin<br>sesame | |
| Animal produce | | unpasteurized<br>    goat's milk<br>    produce | meat<br>poultry<br>fish<br>eggs<br>dairy produce |
| Oils and fats[3] | flaxseed oil<br>hemp oil | olive oil<br>sesame oil<br>sunflower oil<br>walnut oil | refined/<br>    hydrogenated oils<br>    and margarines,<br>    saturated animal fats |

*Figure 1, The acid- or alkaline-forming potential of different foods* (cont.)

| | Alkaline-forming | Mildly acid-forming | Very acid-forming |
|---|---|---|---|
| Sweeteners | | barley malt<br>brown rice malt<br>maple syrup<br>untreated honey | white sugar<br>brown sugar<br>all other refined<br>    sweeteners<br>artificial sweeteners |
| Beverages | herbal teas<br>vegetable juices<br>fruit juices<br>water | grain coffee-<br>    substitutes | tea<br>coffee<br>decaff coffee<br>alcohol |
| Salt | | sea salt | table salt |
| Condiments | | miso<br>tamari<br>soya sauce | vinegar |

refined foods such as sugar and white flour products, all items that contain additives and preservatives, cow's milk produce, artificial sweeteners, tea, coffee and alcohol are the top ten.

However extreme cutting out these preparations may sound, most of them contribute very little nutritional value to the body, if any at all. Food allergies are also associated with the intake of many of these substances and even criminal behaviour has been found to have a dramatic link.[4]

Giving them up may not be an easy task, but attempted gradually they are unlikely to be terribly missed. As with any transition, moving from one set of circumstances to another requires steadfast determination and self-discipline. It's always a good idea to do it little by little, slowly cutting out the baddies and replacing them with the good guys. That way, the body has time to adjust to the changes being made, and there won't be a tremendous rebellion to deal with. And once the temporary cravings and withdrawals have passed and the body has had space to recuperate, a newfound vitality and aliveness will be discovered.

At the end of the day, what is said about one man's medicine being another's poison should always be acknowledged; for some a raw food diet is favourable, others may not fare so well on such a regime. Protein and calorific requirements will also differ from person to person, along with other nutritional needs. And as personal life circumstances change, necessities change too.

Some individuals are allergic to particular nuts, while others have trouble digesting beans. I am even aware of cases where there have been adverse reactions to onions, carrots and other commonly eaten vegetables. As we are all built differently we must listen to our bodies to know what is best. Often this can prove difficult, due to the variety of foods we eat in one day. But as we begin to omit the well-known troublemakers, these idiosyncrasies among normally healthy edibles can be spotted more easily.

It's often not the food itself that's to blame, but our faulty immune systems overreacting to perfectly innocent substances. In time, as we detoxify the body of waste materials and strengthen it through proper nutrition, these adverse responses will begin to disappear.

## GOING ORGANIC

Having sussed out the standards for healthy eating, there's another big step to take before nearing the ultimate nutritional goal. And that's swapping the commercial chemicalization of our food for clean, solid organics.

Ninety-nine per cent of all our produce, unless certified organic, is sprayed with a range of chemical pesticides, amongst others insecticides, fungicides, weedkillers and rat poison. These toxic compounds not only poison our food but can leach into neighbouring crops and rivers, causing damage to both the land and the wildlife that live on it. Some pesticides, together with nitrates from synthetic fertilizers, have even found their way into underground water systems, contaminating our water supply.

Although the Government states that the levels of pesticides used are well within the safety margins, random testing has proved otherwise. Many farmers mix chemicals before spraying, and the combined and cumulative effects of such concoctions are still uncertain.

Research suggests that the build-up of these chemical cocktails in the body, like other poisons, is potentially hazardous and may contribute to the cause of cancerous growths, birth defects and other alarming conditions. And as many species of insects become resistant to these man-made atrocities, other more lethal chemicals, some of which have been banned, are being selected.

So besides peeling or vigorously washing our fruit and veg, which may only remove post-harvest chemicals, it's best to opt for organic, wherever possible. Farmers relying on alternative means to raise their crops apply a combination of safe and environmentally friendly methods of pest control, including harmless insects such as ladybirds that are natural enemies of pests to keep them at bay, crop rotation to prevent pests establishing themselves in fields and companion planting, which involves growing specific species in close proximity for mutual support.

Being free from chemical residues, grown on naturally fertile soil and nurtured with natural composts, organic produce retains its nutrient content and contains more protein, vitamins and minerals than intensively farmed crops. This means it tastes better too. We can also be assured that we'll be avoiding irradiated and genetically engineered foods – other up-and-coming methods of money-manipulating monstrosities.

Going organic may at present be more expensive, but as the demand becomes greater the prices will eventually fall. If we want quality in our lives, then surely paying a little extra for our health and our environment will work out much cheaper in the long run.

# CHAPTER 2

# Foods that Help

*'Let Food be Thy Medicine and Medicine Thy Food'*
— HIPPOCRATES

It's more than 2,000 years since Hippocrates, known to historians as the great father of medicine, taught the foundations of natural health care. A man way ahead of his time, his work has been carried forward to this day and a modern version of his famous oath is still uttered by those beginning medical practice. It is sad, then, to see that such a holistic approach is largely ignored, even ridiculed by our present medical establishment.

Yet whether through suffering, curiosity or genuine interest many individuals have turned to alternative methods of healing as a way of regaining health. And with numerous studies revealing the benefits of a wholefood diet, it seems only logical that food will play an important role as the medicine of the future.

In this chapter, we take a look at the main food groups that form a balanced diet and discover some of the fascinating healing properties many of them possess.

## GRAINS

Since grains play a major role in everyday eating, we shall begin our eco-friendly journey with the cereal family.

Grain cultivation commenced about 10,000 years ago and is the primary source of sustenance and energy for people throughout the world. Grains are versatile and nutritious and in their whole, unadulterated form contain the majority of nutrients needed for survival.

However, whilst grains have fallen on their feet – big time – there seem to be some clashes of opinion about their intake. For instance, devotees in the raw-food establishment seem to feel that to improve its viability the majority of grain should be eaten sprouted. Others, who combine nutrition and anthropology (the study of man and evolution) go with the theory that because grains are a relatively 'new' food group in the evolutionary process (our hunter-gatherer ancestors did not eat grain), they are not designed for the workings of man's digestion.

As far as I – and a great many others in the nutritional field – am concerned, grains are of utmost value within the nutritional jigsaw. Civilizations the globe over have thrived on wholegrains for generations and fail to exhibit any of the trendy torments rife in our up-to-date society.

In the warm months of summer, germinated grains are a most welcome accompaniment, whilst well-simmered cereals throughout the winter are an essential must.

In the past it has always been recommended that grains should be combined with other foods, particularly legumes, to obtain a complete protein. This is because they tend to have lower ratios of certain essential amino acids (protein building-blocks), which decrease the amount of usable protein available. Although traditionally many cultures have obtained their nourishment by this combining ritual, new research suggests that as long as grains are eaten in the context of a wholefood diet there is no need to mix them at the same meal.

Nevertheless, combining grains with their compatible partners, which include beans, pulses and seeds, increases the usable amount of protein by 30 per cent – an important factor when protein needs are considered.

Besides possessing a great variety in the way of nutrition, grains have a particularly profound stabilizing effect on both mind and body. Eaten daily, they allow us to carry out our tasks with enthusiasm and clarity, helping us to strike a balance between the material and spiritual realms of life.

Regrettably, here in the West, as in many parts of the world, most grain is eaten in its white, refined state. Although this process may extend shelf-life, the fibre and most of the nutrients found in the germ and outer husk are removed, leaving us with little more than (nutrientless) empty calories. Processed grains tend to behave more like sugar when ingested, unsettling blood glucose levels and causing cravings and mood swings. It's therefore wise to stick to eating the whole food if any of the benefits are to be retrieved.

Another quandary we have got ourselves into comes from our passion for wheat. Bread and pasta, two of the most popular wheat-based products, are eaten with virtually every meal, leaving other cereals sitting on the shelf. In fact, we've consumed so much of the stuff that wheat allergy and intolerance to gluten (a sticky cereal protein) are extremely common. Matters are made worse by commercial strains of wheat being genetically modified to contain a higher percentage of gluten. This enables bread to turn out larger and lighter, generating increased production from the same amount of raw materials.

As gluten is present in wheat, rye, barley and oats, all four may need to be avoided by those susceptible and substituted with gluten-free grains. These include rice, buckwheat, millet quinoa and amaranth.[1]

Wheat bran is also best avoided due to its high levels of phytate, which latches on to minerals in the digestive system and carries them out of the body. If an all-round wholefood diet is consumed, additional fibre should not be necessary, although rice bran can be resorted to if required.

Want to limit wheat but can't keep away from the bread bin? Then get stuck into spelt and kamut, two ancient strains of wheat that have recently made a comeback.

Those who react quite severely to the ingestion of wheat should first try kamut or spelt in small amounts or else confirm tolerance through kinesiology or other forms of allergy testing.

*Figure 2, The symptoms of wheat allergies and gluten intolerance*

| Wheat allergy | Gluten intolerance |
|---|---|
| runny nose | bloating |
| flu-like manifestations | abdominal pain |
| heart palpitations | diarrhoea |
| oedema | anaemia |
| eczema | weight loss |
| forgetfulness | fatigue |
| depression | depression |
| schizophrenia | |
| (symptoms may vary from person to person) | |

## Spelt

Spelt is an unhybridized cereal from the same genus as common wheat, containing more fibre and up to 30 per cent more protein than its cousin. It also possesses mucopolysaccharides, special carbohydrates that stimulate the immune system. Although some gluten is present, due to its comparative solubility spelt can be endured by most. Spelt bread has an inviting aroma and beats the taste of ordinary wheat-based breads. It's also available in pasta form and as a flour.

## Kamut

Higher in nutrients than today's modern wheat, kamut is an old Egyptian pure-bred strain, particularly appealing to those with wheat sensitivities. Like spelt, kamut does contain gluten, but due to its genetic make-up and rarity in the diet, it proves to be a suitable wheat replacer.

## Grain eating guidelines

- To enhance digestion, chew grains to a pulp.
- Eat grains on a rotating basis, so that allergies are less likely to develop.

- Try not to combine grains with animal or dairy protein, as these food groups are digestively antagonistic.
- Replace the gluten-housing grains in the diet with others.
- Dilute high-protein grains such as quinoa and amaranth with less concentrated cereals such as rice.

### Grain cooking guidelines

Wash the grains well by covering them with 2–3 times the volume of water and swirling them around to remove unwanted particles. Rinse off the water and repeat.

*Figure 3, Grain cooking times and liquid proportions*

| Grain | Amount of grain | Amount of water | Cooking time |
|---|---|---|---|
| Amaranth | 1 cup | 2½ cups | 35 mins |
| Pot barley (soak overnight) | 1 cup | 3 cups | 1 hour |
| Buckwheat (roasted) | 1 cup | 2 cups | 20 mins |
| Bulgar wheat | 1 cup | 2 cups | 12–15 mins |
| Oats – whole (soak overnight) | 1 cup | 2 cups | 1 hour |
| Millet | 1 cup | 3 cups | 45 mins |
| Brown rice | 1 cup | 2 cups | 35 mins |
| Wild rice | 1 cup | 3 cups | 50 mins |
| Wheat berries (soak overnight) | 1 cup | 3 cups | 45 mins |
| Quinoa | 1 cup | 2 cups | 15 mins |

Bring a saucepan with the right amount of water to boil, add the grain and wait until the water starts to re-bubble. Place the saucepan lid on and simmer on a very low flame until all the liquid has been absorbed and the grain is soft. Before removing the saucepan lid, wait 10 minutes; this prevents the grains from becoming sticky. Sea salt may be added at the time of bringing the water to boil but adjusting the palate to salt-free cereals is always encouraged.

Grains can also be pressure cooked, yielding a softer, more concentrated outcome. This cooking practice requires slightly less water than usual and is suitable during the cooler seasons, when extra warmth is needed. Pressure cooking is particularly useful in winter; see page 159.

To round off our Great Grain Guide, here's an insight into some fascinating family facts.

- Short-grain brown rice, when well chewed, is a reliable colon cleanser.
- Drinking the tea made from boiling dried whole corn kernels has been shown to help relieve kidney problems.
- Oats are a wonderful tonic for the brain and nervous system, due to their rich phosphorus content. They also possess powerful cholesterol-busting properties. This is linked to a soluble fibre in oat bran known as beta-glucans, which interferes with the absorption and production of cholesterol.
- Another compound that helps lower high blood-fats is gamma-oryzanol, stored in the outer husk of wholegrain rice.
- Amaranth and quinoa contain all eight essential amino acids and are top-quality forms of protein.
- Quinoa is extremely rich in calcium and iron, making it an excellent substitute for meat and dairy products.
- Millet is the only alkaline-forming member of the true grain family.
- Buckwheat is an excellent source of the bioflavonoid rutin, a substance that helps strengthen the walls of blood capillaries and is naturally anti-inflammatory.
- As a remedy for diarrhoea and fluid retention, barley water, made from the water in which barley has been boiled, can be drunk daily. Barley also contains antiviral and anti-cancer properties.

## LEGUMES

The next food group on our agenda is legumes. Like grains, they are one of the 'newer' foods in man's biological history, yet one of the oldest to be cultivated. They reign second to cereals in importance as a crop and provide the best source of protein in the plant kingdom.

Beans, lentils, peas and (surprisingly) peanuts all belong to the legume family, of which there are over 1,000 different varieties. Besides being rich in protein, legumes are a good source of starch, vitamin B, calcium, magnesium, potassium, phosphorus, iron, zinc and essential fatty acids. The fibre present is of two kinds, soluble and insoluble. While the soluble part works at reducing cholesterol in the body, the insoluble portion helps stabilize blood-sugar levels and promotes bowel function. Lecithin, another factor that has been noted in beans, also helps keep fat levels in check.

Despite the many benefits legumes provide, they've still managed to create a rather troublesome name for themselves. We've all heard the jests and jokes coined about beans and the digestive system, and it's for this reason that they are often avoided. The gassy after-effects are actually created by bacteria in the large intestine, busily at work breaking down oligosaccharides – indigestible starches found more or less in all legumes. And with the clan rich in both protein and starch, the need for appropriate digestive enzymes to be produced at the same time puts a strain on things.

But don't let this be a put-off. Prepared to proper instruction, the after-dinner rebukes of feasting on beans can be greatly reduced. Here are a few ways to savour these morsels and preen them to perfection.

- To help disperse some of the gas-producing compounds in legumes, soak them overnight before cooking. Red lentils are the exception.
- Always discard soak water and rinse the legumes well before cooking.
- Add a few finely cut strips of rehydrated kombu to the saucepan whilst cooking legumes. This provides three positive modes of action: it tenderizes protein, improves flavour and increases nutrient content.
- Fennel, cumin seeds, a few bay leaves and a little ginger are other flavoursome digestion enhancers that can be added during the cooking process.

- Soya and red kidney beans should be quick boiled for 10 minutes before being left to simmer. This releases trypsin inhibitors, which interfere with protein digestion.
- If salt is desired, it should be added towards the end of the cooking period so as not to cause the skin of the legumes to remain tough.
- Ensure that beans are always cooked well. This aids the breakdown process of the starch and improves digestibility.
- Sprouting is another technique that converts legumes into a more easily digestible food. This method is covered in some detail in Chapter 6.

As with all natural foods, legumes also possess therapeutic qualities. Here are a few leguminous legends for you to put to the test.

- For the treatment of kidney and bladder problems, boil adzuki beans in five times as much water for an hour and drink the juice. Repeat daily.
- Consuming the cooking water left from boiling mung beans may be beneficial as a remedy for food poisoning, dysentery, diarrhoea and painful urination.
- Soya beans contain compounds known as phytosterols, which inhibit the uptake of cholesterol by blocking its absorption. Phytosterols also embody oestrogenic properties and function to stabilize oestrogen levels in the system. This is beneficial for women who suffer from premenstrual tension or menopausal symptoms and may help prevent the development of hormone-related cancers.
- The water left from boiling black turtle beans has shown to be effective for alleviating kidney stones, laryngitis and hot flushes.

## VEGETABLES

Whilst grains and beans are building foods, the nature of most vegetables is more eliminative. This is linked to their rich fluid and fibre content, coupled with a high alkaline-forming ash.

Vegetables are abundant in a number of vitamins and minerals, including the four main electrolytes: calcium, magnesium, sodium and potassium. They are also one of the best sources of antioxidants and contain potent plant compounds, known as phytochemicals, that serve to protect us from the exposure to damaging elements.

Seaweed, often neglected in the Western diet, is a delicious edible that falls into the vegetable category. Don't be dissuaded by their often unappealing front: sea vegetables have some wonderful flavours that can enhance an assortment of dishes and provide utmost nutrition.

Because different vegetables grow in different climates and seasons, they can assist us in acclimatizing to our environment. It's for this reason that it's important to eat only those vegetables that are seasonal and locally grown. To make this a little clearer, vegetables that appear naturally in the warmer months or grow in hot regions tend to have a thinning effect on the blood and make a lighter contribution to our system. Winter or cold climate vegetables, on the other hand, like parsnips, swede and potatoes, are starchier and more filling and create inner warmth. By eating vegetables that are in season we can adjust smoothly to each turn of the calendar and stand a better chance of maintaining good health.

Although vegetables are exceptionally good for us, there are some that contain small amounts of naturally occurring toxins, and need to be treated with a little care. Firstly, plants that contain oxalic acid, such as spinach, swiss chard, kale and beet tops, should be limited in the diet of those with poor calcium metabolism – for example, those with osteoarthritis; osteoporosis, those prone to kidney stones or other ailments in which there is abnormal hardening of the bone. Oxalic acid depletes calcium from the body by blocking its absorption and can damage the kidneys by depositing calcium oxalate crystals in the urinary tract. Fortunately, much of the oxalate can be removed by quick blanching or boiling these greens. Secondly, turnips, cabbage and mustard contain goitrogens which block how the body uses iodine. However, once they are cooked these substances are inactivated.

A final toxin that aggravates certain conditions, particularly arthritis, is found in the class of foods known as nightshades. These include tomatoes, aubergine, peppers (with the exception of the black variety) and to a lesser degree, potatoes. Nightshade plants contain strong alkaloids which when eaten regularly may weaken the system.

But don't panic. Potatoes and tomatoes, top of the crops in the West, can be continued to be consumed quite safely, providing they are eaten in moderate amounts (eg one serving twice a week), in conjunction with a wholefood diet. However potatoes that are tinged with green must be avoided.

Whereas processed or artificial 'foods' are not good for us (full stop), the groups of vegetables I have just mentioned, being natural contain countless positive attributes. Therefore, if treated wisely, they pose no problem to healthy individuals.

### A *personal endeavour*

When it comes to harmless ways of eating one's fill, fresh fruit and vegetables definitely come tops. Besides exercising four to five times a week, to maintain a relatively fatless figure, I always ensure that there are plenty of fruit and vegetables waiting for me when I arrive home.

In the spring and summer, I chop up a huge bowl of mixed salad, enough to last a couple of days. This may not be the ideal way of preserving vitamins and minerals, but at least I know when hunger strikes I'll be delving into the salad dish and not the biscuit tin. During the winter, I prepare a large vat of home-made soup and store it in the fridge for the following day. I also check there's plenty of colourful roots and greens, ready to pop into the steamer.

The motto here is: one can never eat too many vegetables! Together with grains, they should be the central feature of every main meal.

# FRUIT

Naturally ripened by the sun, fruit is packed with nature's goodness. It's highly cleansing and alkalizing (except for cranberries, prunes and rhubarb,[2] which contain benzoic and oxalic acid) and can be eaten to enhance the elimination of toxins. Care should be taken with citrus fruits, though, as they can be overly detoxifying and may cause reactions.

Generally fruits contain more vitamins than vegetables whereas vegetables rate higher in the mineral stakes. They're also a rich source of natural sugars, live enzymes and powerful plant pigments that work as antioxidants. As our bodies digest this food batch relatively quickly (within half an hour), they're best eaten away from heavier foods, to prevent fermentation. Between meals is probably a good time to fit them in. The exception to the rule is acid fruits (see page 98) with nuts and seeds, which seem to combine reasonably well.

Fruit juices are preferable when diluted with water to reduce the amount of fructose (fruit sugar) present. This will help curb blood-sugar fluctuations, as fruit juices, not remaining intact with the whole food, are often rather concentrated.

Because the growth of fruit, like vegetables, is governed by climate, they should only be eaten when in season. Summer and early autumn seem to be the ideal times to indulge, when there's an abundance of cooling and refreshing varieties available. In the colder seasons, fruit should be eaten sparingly as it can be too chilling and eliminative for the winter cycle. Cooked or dried fruit is a better option at this time. Consuming tropical fruits such as mangos and kiwis in a temperate zone, however delectable and healthy they look, is also not a good idea. Such fruits may actually weaken the system if eaten regularly and increase the risk of allergies.

# NUTS AND SEEDS

In a nutshell, nuts and seeds contain the potential for supporting an entire plant. So imagine the nourishment that's locked into these compact little fellows. Whilst both possess admirable amounts of protein, vitamins B and E and plenty of the finest fats, seeds win when it comes to the mineral count.

Nuts are best purchased in their hard shells, which protect them from oxygen, light and heat, a trio of factors which hasten their rancidity. Alternatively, nuts, like seeds, should be obtained from a reputable store with a high turnover, and once opened kept sealed in the fridge.

Avoid commercially prepared roasted and salted nuts as they are overly rich in salt and fat. Nuts that have been ground or chopped should also be given a miss as they oxidize quicker. It's far better to chop or grind freshly bought nuts at home, whenever they're required.

For those who are especially sensitive or allergic, here's a few titbits to watch out for in the province of nuts.

Special attention should be taken when eating peanuts, as they can easily become contaminated with moulds that produce a carcinogenic substance called aflatoxin.[3] In large amounts aflatoxin can damage the liver, and although rare can cause death. For this reason peanuts are best purchased in their shells and avoided by those with allergies, liver problems, yeast infections and degenerative diseases. Peanuts can also cause skin outbreaks.

Those who have a sensitive disposition should also be cautious of cashews, due to the presence of naturally occurring caustic oil. This irritating substance is usually removed once the nuts have been skinned, but to ensure their safety they can be lightly roasted.

Another no-no is aimed at anyone who suffers from any form of herpes condition. This is because nuts contain high levels of the amino acid arginine, which when combined with their low lysine content may trigger the virus to become active.

Given their high fat and calorie content, nuts and seeds should be eaten in moderation. They're delicious sprinkled in home-made mueslis, salads and desserts or can simply be enjoyed as a snack. Nut and seed butters also make appetizing spreads but must always be checked for their freshness and signs of rancidity.

Here are some Nutty Notions and Seedy Snippets to consider:

- Almonds are reputed for their anti-cancer compound amygdalin, also known as laetrile or vitamin $B_{17}$. Jason Winters, author of *Killing Cancer* (Vinten Press), advises eating ten almonds a day as part of a cancer-prevention plan. Almonds also possess therapeutic levels of salicylate, a natural pain-killing agent.
- As a folk remedy for chronic coughs and bronchitis, chew steamed chestnuts. They are also beneficial when ground up in their raw state and applied externally to sores.
- Pine nut kernels are useful as a lubricant for the lungs and intestines.
- Brazil nuts are high in the mineral selenium, a powerful antioxidant often lacking in many foods.
- The rich levels of vitamin B and manganese found in walnuts make them an excellent brain food. In fact, their two-lobed appearance even resembles that of a human brain. Walnuts also have the benefit of containing ellagic acid – an antioxidant and cancer fighter.
- The bountiful zinc and essential fatty acid content found in pumpkin seeds makes them an excellent food for the prevention and treatment of prostate problems in men. A small handful eaten daily is recommended.
- Pumpkin seeds are also an effective remedy for dispelling intestinal worms. Combine three tablespoons of seeds with half a small onion and a cup of soya milk and liquidize in a blender. Take this mixture three times a day for five days.
- To prevent or clear constipation, take one heaped tablespoon of linseed twice a day, with plenty of water.
- Hemp seeds contain 45 per cent of their nutrient value in protein and hold the best balance of essential fatty acids over any other food.

## FATS AND OILS

Getting the facts right about fats can be confusing, especially when we're constantly bombarded by the 'low-fat' hype. Yes it's true, our diets should be low in fat – the bad fat, that is. But there are certain fats, known as essential fatty acids, that play a vital role in the health and proper functioning of many internal processes and a lack of them can result in a number of disturbances.

There are two prime kinds of essential fatty acids, linoleic acid (omega 6) and alpha linolenic acid (omega 3) and from these all other fats that we need can be made. Good sources of linoleic acid include seeds, nuts, beans, grains and vegetables. Alpha linolenic acid is a little more scarce, but the major suppliers are hemp, flax and pumpkin seeds, walnuts, soya beans and dark leafy greens. For non-vegetarians, oily fish such as sardines, mackerel and salmon also contain these oils, although how infiltrated they are by sea pollution is a big question.

In nature, there are also certain foods that help to dissolve the bad fats in the body. These include lecithin-rich beans (lecithin being an effective emulsifier), and some of the stronger-tasting vegetables, including radish, daikon, onion, leek, garlic and turnip. Organic cold-pressed flax- or hempseed oil also works at diminishing the negative fats, whilst supplying both omega 3 and omega 6 essential fatty acids.

## The types of fats

In nature there are three main types of fats: saturated, mono-saturated and polyunsaturated.

### Saturated

Saturated fats are solid or semi-solid at room temperature and are largely of animal origin, such as butter and lard; the exceptions are coconut, palm and palm kernel oils. Saturated fats found in meat, dairy produce, tropical oils, fried food and hydrogenated and partially hydrogenated vegetable oils are closely linked to the increased risk of most degenerative conditions. They are unnecessary and are best omitted from the diet.

*Monounsaturated*

Monounsaturated fats are liquid at room temperature, but if refrigerated will thicken. Olive, avocado, sesame and several nut oils fit into this niche. Whilst in their whole form they are extremely nourishing, most do not show any great health-enhancing benefits. The exception is extra-virgin (cold-pressed) olive oil, which helps reduce low-density lipoprotein (LDL), vehicles that carry fats and cholesterol into the blood and cells. It also aids the increase of the good high-density lipoprotein (HDL) fats.

*Polyunsaturated*

Polyunsaturated fats remain liquid both at room temperature and when refrigerated. They possess essential fatty acids.

Ideally, fats are best consumed in their whole, natural state, where they are found together with other symbiotic nutrients, including fat-soluble vitamins, lecithin and antioxidants, that help protect them.

**Vegetable oils**

*Unrefined*

Extracted plant oils should only be taken in their most natural form; ensure that the word 'unrefined' is clearly stated on the bottle. These include flax, sunflower, safflower, soya, pumpkin, hemp and walnut oil. Extra-virgin olive and sesame are also placed in this group, although being monounsaturated rather than polyunsaturated they lack essential fatty acids.

Unrefined plant oils have been mechanically expelled under relatively low temperatures and if stored properly retain much of their goodness.

*Refined*

Refined vegetable oils should not be used for any purpose. The light-coloured ones found in supermarkets and grocers have all been extracted by the application of heat and harsh chemicals. All nutrients are depleted and the heating process causes some of the oil to be converted from its natural cis-fatty acid state to form trans-fatty acids, synthetic fats that have the same negative impact as fats represented by meat and dairy. They cause fatty deposits to build up in the arteries and increase the risk of the development of a range of chronic ills.

*Figure 4, The wrong fats and the right fats and what they do*

| What the wrong fats do | What the right fats do |
|---|---|
| raise blood fat levels | inhibit abnormal cell multiplication |
| clog up the circulatory system | help maintain normal blood pressure |
| block digestive and liver function | check cholesterol synthesis |
| retard skin quality | prevent the blood from becoming sticky |
| create hormone imbalances | balance hormones |
| encourage weight gain and mental and physical sluggishness | reinforce the immune system |
|  | reduce inflammation |
|  | aid the removal of excess body fluid |
|  | regulate nerve function |
|  | promote mental and physical health |

## Fat and oil cooking guidelines

When it comes to sautéing and stir-frying, extra-virgin olive oil is probably the most appropriate choice, with sesame on the shortlist. Whilst being low in the health-destroying saturates, they are relatively stable when exposed to heat, and have a fairly high smoke point.

Besides olive and sesame (and peanut if it can be found), unrefined oils should *never* be heated. This is because they have a low smoke threshold and being heat sensitive cause molecules to react once disclosed. These oils are fine ingredients for salad dressings, dips and other raw administrations.

A safer way to stir-fry, causing the least damage to the cooking oil, is to add the ingredients to the pan before the oil starts to sizzle. Another method is to place a little water in the saucepan before adding the oil. This prevents the temperature from rising too high, thus avoiding the danger of allowing the oil to overheat.

As for deep-frying, this method of cooking is potentially hazardous and should certainly be avoided. Exposing oil to the combination of light, oxygen and extremely hot temperatures produces unstable molecules and toxic compounds that are precursors of disease. Regularly eating food that has been cooked in this way is one of the most efficient means of damaging body cells, and the cumulative effects over the years contribute greatly to the ageing process. If deep-frying food is an occasional imperative, then let it be a rare treat – and treat it with respect.

Five ways to ensure your oil doesn't spoil.

- Purchase unrefined oils in dark-coloured bottles so that they are protected from surrounding light.
- Only buy oils that are stored in glass bottles. Those that are packaged in plastic may combine with the synthetic material to form toxic plasticides.
- Once open, store oils (with the exception of olive) in the fridge, to slow down the oxidation process.
- Never re-use an oil once it has been heated.
- When heating an oil, do not allow it to get so hot that it begins to smoke.

If we insist on using some kind of fat as a spreading agent, then we have to decide whether butter or margarine is more fitting.

For those who want to stick with butter, choose the organic, unsalted varieties.

For those who prefer margarine, the unhydrogenated, water-based ones available from health food stores will suffice. Freshness must always be ensured and such margarines, like most unrefined oils, must not be heated. All other commercial margarines should be avoided. As with refined oils, they contain trans-fatty acids and interfere with the proper utilization of the essential fats in the diet.

As alternatives to both butter and margarine, try nut or seed spreads, or like the Mediterraneans, a dribble of olive oil.

# WATER

So far, there has been much said about food – but nothing yet mentioned about water. Water, of course, like the air we breathe, is one of our most important lifelines. Our bodies are made up of almost 70 per cent of it and it's the medium in which all cellular reactions take place. Without sufficient amounts, nutrients and chemical messengers cannot fully reach their destinations, and toxins and waste products cannot be efficiently carried away. Dr Batmanghelidj, author of *The Body's Many Cries For Water* (Global Health Solutions), shows through extensive research that it's a lack of water in the body that causes the manifestation of many disease states. He also demonstrates that most of these conditions can be astoundingly improved just by correcting this shortage.

Most of us don't drink nearly enough water. We have become so parched and dehydrated that even our thirst signals have packed up. The need for water is often confused with hunger or temporarily suppressed with regular cups of coffee, tea or sweetened sodas.

Caffeinated or sweetened liquids do not increase our fluid levels. Being powerful diuretics, they actually drain the body of fluid and create a continual internal crisis.

Every day, we lose about 2 litres (3½ pints/9C) of water through our kidneys, lungs, bowel and skin. To account for this loss, we need to drink every day a minimum of 1.5–2 litres/2½–3½ pints (UK)/6¼–9C (US) of water. Extra is required if the weather is hot and during and after exercise.

Other fluids that sustain our health, such as fruit and vegetable juices, herbal teas, grain coffees and the water found in whole, natural food, can add to this intake. To hydrate ourselves properly we must also refrain from taking tea, coffee, soft drinks and alcohol.

Drinking plenty of water every day is all very well, but knowing what water to drink is another matter. Tap water, in the majority of areas, is definitely out. Most supplies have been tainted with numerous contaminants, including nitrates from fertilizers, pesticides, bacteria, heavy metals, chlorine and even radioactive waste.

So if we can't drink the water from our own kitchen sink, what are our options?

Bottled water is an expensive alternative, the quality of it varying greatly. Although water doesn't react with plastic in the way that oil does, glass bottles are preferable because they can be recycled. As water is a global substance it doesn't matter too much where it comes from as long as it's of a high quality. If spring or mineral water is the preference, go for the ones that are low in nitrates, sodium and other minerals. Although minerals are crucial in our diets, those that are found in water have come straight from a rock surface and have not yet been absorbed via a plant, so they remain inorganic and cannot be utilized. Inorganic minerals present in water have been found to cause hardening in soft tissues of the body and are potentially destructive.

## Jug filters

Jug filter cartridges contain activated carbon and ion exchange resins and can siphon up to 150 litres (33 UK gallons/40 US gallons) of water. They reduce a percentage (depending on the brand) of the chlorine, pesticides, heavy metals and bacteria, and some also reduce nitrates. Although jug filters are silverized to prevent bacteria build-up, it's recommended that cartridges are renewed once a month.

## Distillers

Distillation units work via a boiling, cooling method and require a fair amount of electricity to do the job. Despite this, almost all impurities and inorganic minerals are eradicated.

## Reverse osmosis

This system comes as a plumbed-in filter that fits under the sink. It operates by an 'under pressure' technique, pushing the water through a semi-permeable membrane, whilst separating it from unwanted molecules. Reverse osmosis removes toxic metals, pesticide residues, nitrates, bacteria, chlorine and hard-water minerals.

# CHAPTER 3

# Foods that Hinder

In Chapter 2 we ventured into the spheres where food has a predominantly positive impact upon our health. Here we move on into the darker closets of nutrition – or lack of it – and glean some of the more detrimental substances that are commonly consumed in our day-to-day dining.

So as not to make it all too tiresome, the food groups, or 'substances' as they are more appropriately described, and the threats they pose, are covered in short, simple points. And to make it easier to wave farewell to some of these fake allies, plenty of healthy alternatives have been laid down.

## WHERE TO START

Knowing where to start and what to kick off with, whilst putting this segment together, proved to be a minor distraction. Should sugar be the first to bite the bullet or should it be meat to take the plunge? To lend a helping hand, I've enlisted the assistance of two Oriental friends – namely 'yin' and 'yang'.

For those who are not yet familiar with this complementary couple, here's a brief introduction. Basically yin (expansive) and yang (contractive) are two opposing forces that exist in all things. If we look around us, we can see them at play. For example, day and night, hot and cold, winter and summer, male and female, and so on. In reality, these forces are actually one, but, like a coin that has two sides, manifest duality.

It was Japanese-born George Ohsawa who first applied the ancient concept of 'yin' and 'yang' to nutrition. By healing himself of a terminal illness, Ohsawa was able to work out that when a food is relatively uniform or moderate in either 'yin' or 'yang', as it is in most wholefoods, the body can return to and remain in good health. If the foods consumed possess qualities that are extreme in either energy, sickness and disease will eventually prevail. Ohsawa coined this dietary philosophy 'macrobiotics' and after much study, brought his teachings to the West.

To gain a clearer image of 'yin' and 'yang' in relation to diet, please refer to figure 5. Notice that the items listed in the moderate categories form part of a healthy diet. Those in the extreme ones upset the body's natural equilibrium and for the most part are forbidden territory.

*Figure 5, The 'yin' and 'yang' classifications of different foods*

| Extremely yin | Moderately yin | Moderately yang | Extremely yang |
|---|---|---|---|
| sugar | vegetables | wholegrains | meat |
| chocolate | sprouted grains | legumes | fish |
| refined foods | local fruit and fruit | root vegetables | eggs |
| artificial | and vegetable | sourdough bread | salt |
| sweeteners | juices | seeds | hard, salty cheese |
| most dairy produce | tofu | nuts | |
| other-climate fruit | tempeh | miso | |
| spices | soya milk | tamari | |
| tea | vegetable oils | | |
| coffee | natural sweeteners | | |
| soft drinks | | | |
| alcohol | | | |

To stay with the macrobiotic way of thinking, this chapter is placed under two main headings, 'Yin' and 'Yang'. Although the inclusion of an Eastern concept into a book that's based around temperate-climate eating may seem a little contradictory, on the whole, macrobiotics tailors to fit in with 'local' diets and is therefore universal in application. For this reason it has proven to be a highly successful practice all over the world.

## THE YIN EXTREME

As illustrated in figure 5, the preparations that cause us to become overly 'yin', or 'yinned out', generally include sugar, stimulants, refined grain products and dairy foods. Too many yin foods in the diet can lead to the following tendencies:

*Figure 6, The effects of an excess of yin foods*

| Physical | Mental/Emotional |
|---|---|
| headaches (frontal) | lack of self-confidence |
| fatigue | oversensitivity |
| muscle aches | confusion |
| easy bruising | scattered thinking |
| respiratory difficulties | loss of will-power |
| varicose veins | fear |
| cystitis | suspicion |
| asthma | schizophrenia |
| diabetes | |
| hypoglycaemia | |

### Sugar

To begin with, let's look on the yin side of what's what with a universal favourite. It's found lurking in everything from cakes, cookies and ice cream to curries, convenience meals and ketchup; that sweet but not so innocent tease, sugar.

The term sugar can refer to one of two things.

A 'complex' carbohydrate is where the sugar is found intact in its whole, natural state, eg inside a piece of fruit, together with fibre and other nutriments. This type of sugar is broken down slowly in the digestive tract and absorbed into the bloodstream at a steady pace, helping to maintain blood-sugar balance.

A 'simple' carbohydrate unless it has been naturally broken down by way of sprouting or fermentation, is a sugar that has been extracted from its original source, and therefore becomes highly refined. A simple sugar enters the bloodstream far too quickly for the body to handle, so much of it is converted into an energy reserve or stored as fat.

On average we consume between 30 and 35 teaspoons of refined sugar every day. In its unprocessed state that would mean having to chew our way through about 90 feet of sugar cane. And don't believe that the brown stuff is much better – because it's not. It's just white crystals that have been coloured with molasses, the liquid syrup drained from the refining industry. Some of the conditions excess sugar intake has been linked to are dental caries, hypoglycaemia, diabetes, fungal infections (eg *Candida albicans* and thrush), obesity, poor immune function, cataracts, fatigue, raised blood fats, heart disease, cancer and mental disorders.[1]

So here goes. Exposed are some of the reasons why we should think twice about entertaining sugar and the hordes of refined food items that contain it in our diet.

Sugar
- is devoid of all vitamins, minerals, protein, fat and fibre yet laden with calories.
- eats up stored nutrients from the body, to aid its assimilation.
- triggers cravings for more sugar and the desire for salt and meat.
- invokes a feeling of constant hunger, due to its lack of stable nourishment.
- is highly acid-forming.
- causes drastic fluctuations in blood-glucose levels and wears out the pancreas and adrenal glands, which toil to try and correct the imbalance.

The following are some of the more natural sweeteners available. It must be remembered though that all sweeteners besides fresh fruit are highly concentrated and should only be used in small amounts.

*Grain malt syrups*

Brown rice, maize and barley malt syrups are natural sugars developed from whole cereals. The grains are allowed to sprout and the enzymes that are produced from this process convert the starch into sugars. Through further fermentation, grain syrups are manufactured. Besides being one third the sweetness of white sugar, unlike refined sweeteners that steal stored nourishment from the body they contain the necessary nutrients required for their metabolism.

*Honey*

Processed by bees from plant nectar, high-standard honey contains small amounts of nutrients and is a viable cane replacer. Refrain from buying impure products, choosing raw, cold-pressed versions from specialized food shops or direct from an accredited bee-keeper.

*Maple syrup*

Maple sap, or syrup as we know it, is expressed from the bark of the maple tree. There are different ranks, depending on quality, but generally the lighter coloured concentrates classed as grade 'A' are considered superior. The finest of syrup is well worth the expense. Avoid the cheaper commercial brands as they are likely to be combined with sugary water and other meagre substitutes.

*Amazake*

Amazake is a fermented sweet rice made from cooking the wholegrain with water and koji, a special yeast culture. The enzymes in the koji convert the starch in the cereal to a more digestible carbohydrate, where the mixture begins to resemble a very sweet rice pudding. Being fermented, amazake can replace the need for alcohol in rich fruit cakes and also makes a delicious filling or topping for other desserts. Millet and oat amazakes are also available.

## Stevia

Credited by the Japanese as being the sweetener of the future, stevia has the benefits of being unrefined, virtually free of calories and comparatively nutritious. Taken from the leaves and flower buds of a shrubby Brazilian plant, it seems to be well tolerated by those with blood-sugar disturbances, allergies and problems associated with candida.

## Fructooligosaccharides (FOS)

FOS are non-digestible compounds that have been extracted from various fruit and vegetables. Although they look – and even taste – like white sugar crystals, they are actually quite different and cannot be digested by the human system. Instead they are broken down in the large intestine by certain microflora, producing beneficial organic acids that promote the multiplication of friendly bacteria. FOS also have a positive effect on the blood-sugar level and aid cholesterol reduction.

## Carob

The healthier option to chocolate, carob bean powder is free of caffeine and theobromine, two stimulants found in cocoa. In combination with other sweeteners it lends a richness to baked goods and is ideal for any recipe that calls for chocolate.

## Dried fruit purées

Dried fruit purées can be easily prepared at home by simmering the fruit of choice in three times as much water or fruit juice until all the liquid has been absorbed. Cooking dates in this way converts them into a ready-to-use paste, whilst others such as apricots and raisins may need to be briefly blended.

*Others*

Sugar-free jams, fresh fruit and fruit juice concentrates are other simple sweeteners, ideal for sugaring up cereals, crumbles and pies.

## Dairy produce

Of all the foods that aren't particularly good for us, dairy produce, with cheese at the forefront, seems to be the hardest of preparations to resist. But there are many reasons why cow's milk and its products should be banished from our eating plan. For a start, milk produced by a cow is suited to the needs of a growing calf – and not a human being. By taking a vigilant look at its constituents we can properly begin to wise up to this 'food' faction. Here are a few pointers to help re-evaluate existing beliefs.

Cow's milk
- contains three times as much protein and four times as much calcium as human breast milk – far over the top for a human's nutritional requirements.
- has a high calcium to magnesium ratio, making it difficult for the calcium to be properly employed. Instead of the calcium being absorbed into its needful sites, such as bones and teeth, it may get dumped into soft-tissue areas, causing calcium deposits and abnormal tissue hardening.
- lacks fibre and is full of cholesterol and saturated fat.
- presents lactose, a sugar which cannot be digested by the majority of adults. This is due to a lack of the lactose-digesting enzyme, which normally disappears once we are weaned. Symptoms of lactose intolerance include bloating, gas, stomach cramps and diarrhoea.
- is extremely mucus-forming and clogs up the system, creating a sticky environment in which bacteria prosper.

- is in possession of xanthine oxidase, an enzyme that has been noted to attack the lining of artery walls.
- from non-organic cattle is swarming with antibiotics, growth hormones and pesticide residues, ingested from contaminated feed.

The consumption of milk and its by-products is associated with the following ailments: asthma, arthritis, allergies, diabetes, eczema, fibroids, premenstrual syndrome, kidney stones, multiple sclerosis (MS), Crohn's disease, hardening of the arteries and various forms of cancer.

Many people worry that if they give up dairy foods they will not obtain enough calcium, but since the calcium in milk is not utilized efficiently it is therefore, unlike what we are constantly told, not a reputable supply. To put readers' minds at rest, there are plenty of plant-based calcium sources that can be inserted into the daily diet. These include dark leafy greens, soya preparations, sea vegetables, sesame, pumpkin and sunflower seeds and dried figs.

There are many alternatives to cow's milk.

### Goat's milk produce

For those who do not wish to cut out milky foods altogether, small amounts of organic goat's milk produce can be substituted. Goat's milk is easier to digest than milk from a cow as its protein and fat molecules are more finely distributed. It also poses a smaller chance of triggering allergies.

### Dairy-free substitutes

These days, there's a replacement for just about everything in the dairy cabinet. Soya, rice and oat milk are wholesome options to commercial milk – minus all the bad stuff. There's also some delicious soya-based alternatives for hard and soft cheese, yoghurt, butter and cream.

*Home-made nut milks*

To prepare an ambrosial drink, combine 1 part nuts, eg almonds, cashews or hazelnuts, with 3 parts water and blend until smooth.

## Spices

In the right amounts, adding spice to food can jazz up all sorts of recipes. As we all know, in tropical countries they are well established in traditional meals, where they are believed to enhance digestion.

But beware of the stronger seasonings, especially cayenne pepper and hot chilies, members of the nightshade family. Besides blotting out the more subtle flavours of a meal, they irritate the delicate linings of the digestive tract, causing inflammation and pain. Many Indian clients have complained to me of this and find that the effects become worse when they continue to eat their local diet in a temperate climate.

Milder spices such as paprika, coriander and cumin and sweet spices like nutmeg, cinnamon and ginger are more acceptable in cooler regions. One way of benefiting from the flavour of chilli, without actually ingesting it, is to add a fresh uncut green capsicum to the cooking pot, and remove it before serving.

## Coffee

Another bad boy on the 'yin' hit list is coffee. Highly habit forming, abusive and detrimental to health – what more needs to be said about this lethal-laced beverage? As well as a high caffeine content, coffee also possesses dozens of other harsh components that are responsible for an array of disastrous effects. Drinking decaff coffee is not much worthier, as the caffeine is often removed by way of chemical solvents, and the other unwanted properties are still retained. Here's the expresso run-down on why we shouldn't drink it.

Coffee
- is a temporary stimulant, usually followed by fatigue.
- is addictive, resulting in withdrawal symptoms such as headaches and the 'jitters' when suddenly omitted.
- causes nervousness and confusion.
- raises blood pressure and heart rate.
- increases blood coagulation.
- provokes fatty acids and glucose to be released from the cells into the blood.
- aggravates blood-sugar levels.
- damages chromosomes inside body cells.
- interferes with normal sleep patterns.
- acidifies body tissues.
- blocks the absorption of many vitamins and minerals, including calcium, iron and zinc; there's also a definite link between coffee intake, calcium loss and osteoporosis.
- stimulates acid secretion in the stomach, provoking the potential for stomach ulcers.
- is a powerful diuretic, elevating internal dehydration.
- has a laxative effect and may cause diarrhoea.

Drinking one to five cups of coffee a day can raise the risk of heart disease by up to 60 per cent. More than six cups of coffee increases the chance by 120 per cent. Coffee intake has also been linked to miscarriages and stomach, pancreatic and bladder cancer. There are many healthy alternatives.

*Grain coffee substitutes*

Produced from cereals, roots and fruits, grain coffee substitutes provide much of the flavour and satisfaction of coffee beans without the presence of caffeine and co. They may take a little adjusting to, but once coffee has been kept away from for a few weeks, there'll be no turning back. Like the 'real' thing, they're available in regular and instant varieties and can be drunk both black or white.

*Root coffee substitutes*

Ground, roasted chicory root, an ingredient often found in grain coffee, is very pleasant drunk on its own. Dandelion coffee, prepared from roasted ground dandelion root, is another faithful option.

## Tea

A further substance that has made its fame amongst the millions is tea. Fermented from the less intoxicating green tea leaves, the common cup of *cha* (black tea) possesses almost as much caffeine as a cup of coffee. Tannic acid, which interferes with the uptake of vitamins $B_1$ and $B_{12}$ and theophylline, is an additional disagreeable present that also exerts a similar response. The effects of tea drinking on our health are similar to those of coffee.

As alternatives there's a massive selection of herbal infusions to choose from, from the very basic of aromas to the wild and wonderful. The majority of herbal teas are tannin- and caffeine-free and many contribute a range of therapeutic benefits.[2] To find out how to make a medicinal or herbal tea, turn to page 95.

As an initiation, here are six of the best.

*Camomile*

A firm favourite, camomile's mildness and rich mineral content calms the entire system. It's dependable for easing stomach aches and digestive problems, headaches, nervousness and insomnia.

*Dandelion*

Whilst the root of the dandelion makes a favourable replacement for coffee, the leaves of the plant are often drunk as a medicine.

Dandelion is a powerful diuretic, eliminating water retention caused by fluid build-up. But unlike conventional water tablets that cheat the body of potassium, dandelion is rich in this mineral, ensuring its maintenance. The herb also helps detoxify the blood and liver and is a good one to include when launching into a cleanse.

### Elderflower

This summery scented herb is an effective tea for treating colds and weaknesses of the respiratory tract, including hay fever, sinusitis and catarrhal conditions. For acute symptoms, for instance when hay fever strikes, it can be drunk up to six times a day throughout susceptible periods.

### Fennel

Reminiscent of aniseed, the aroma of fennel tea brings back those childhood sweet-time memories. It's an excellent herb for treating intestinal gas, colic and gout and is also a gentle diuretic.

### Lemon verbena

Sharp and refreshing, lemon verbena is a nice night-time tea, for evening unwinding. It also stimulates digestion, strengthens the nerves and comes to the rescue of feverish colds.

### Nettle

This is one herb tea that I always keep a packet of in the kitchen cupboard. Nettle has a strong green-like but pleasing flavour and is an excellent source of iron. It's also one of those plants that has a myriad of uses. Indications include mild asthma, rheumatism, skin problems, cystitis, anaemia and enlarged prostate – to name but a few.

## Oriental teas

Other teas that have proved to be beneficial are those popular on the macrobiotic scene. These include Kukicha and Mu. Kukicha is an exotic tea brewed from the roasted twigs of the bancha plant. It's the perfect accompaniment to a grain-based diet, aiding the digestion of carbohydrates, and is also known to fortify blood flow. Mu was originally developed by 'Mr Macro' George Ohsawa himself. It is a spicy mix, a blend of 16 different mountain-grown herbs. Mu is good for the circulation, and is indicated in cases of wheezing and breathing difficulties.

## Alcohol

Although there are reports suggesting that alcohol, in moderation, is some kind of boon, other studies disregard these findings. There may be certain isolated properties in specific alcoholic beverages that exert some benefits, but these are swiftly nullified when the entire picture is viewed.

Alcohol is not a drink – it's a drug. In the short term it destroys brain cells, unbalances the blood-sugar level, increases gut permeability, incapacitates immunity and robs the body of a spectrum of nutrients.

Regular consumption of alcohol over the years, even within reason, rots the liver, induces memory loss, deranges the nervous system, increases the risk of breast and other cancers and adversely agitates every cell in the entire system.

## Alternatives

Besides amazake, which can replace alcohol in desserts, there is no substitute for this alien substance. It's well advised to give the bottle the boot, the wine a wave and the beer a bye-bye – for good.

## THE YANG EXTREME

If we glance back at figure 6 on page 31, we can refresh our minds of the items that rest in the 'yang' department. Over-consuming extreme yang foods, such as animal produce and salt, elicits inclinations that are very much the opposite of a yin-based diet.

*Figure 7, The effects of an excess of yang foods*

| Physical | Mental/Emotional |
| --- | --- |
| dry skin | stubbornness |
| muscle tightness and tension | rigidity of mind |
| constipation | quick temper |
| gout | arrogance |
| arthritis | greed |
| high blood pressure | lack of sensitivity towards others |
| hardening of the arteries | materialism |

### Meat

When I was a young girl, vegetarianism was deemed rather odd and promoting an understanding of the 'whys' and 'whats' of such a diet was a lonely battle. Thankfully, these days, I meet like-minded citizens wherever I go and abstaining from flesh is a mushrooming normality.

No one knows for sure why man began to eat his fellow creatures. One theory is that during changing climatic conditions, when plant food was less abundant, animals were consumed as a way to survive. But whilst our forerunners supplemented a mainly plant-based diet with animal produce, people of the present supplement a mainly meat-based diet with plants. In addition, animals are no longer left to roam wild and free in their natural habitat. On the contrary, they are just another consumer item on the conveyor belt, reaching the dining table dead, disfigured and disguised.

To discuss this topic a little more fully, I would like to divide the cons of flesh eating into three distinct sections.

## Biological

I believe that originally we were all vegetarian. Biologically, the human frame has not evolved to digest flesh. If we compare our physiological structure with that of a carnivore, and then with that of a plant-eating animal, we will find that we have a lot more in common with the herbivorous species.

Unlike meat-devouring animals, we do not produce powerful protein-splitting enzymes, essential for the breakdown of this condensed nutrient. Neither do we possess sharp teeth or claws to help us with the unsavoury act. And whilst a carnivore has a short intestine, which allows fast-decaying food to pass through quickly, our own is distinguishingly long. Such an extended canal is suited not to the high putrefactive factors found in meat, but to the rich fibrous and starchy materials that exist in vegetation.

## Moral/ethical

Every time we engage in the eating of animals, we participate in a chain of events instigated by crime. Besides the thousands of animals that are prematurely murdered every day to satisfy selfish stomachs, we also encourage a squad of other violations.

A large proportion of all grain and soya that is grown in the United States goes into feeding livestock, whilst millions of people in the world are dying from starvation. There's also mass wastage of energy, water and fuel in the procedure, plus large-scale damage to surrounding land.

It's easy to close our eyes to the whole issue and pretend that everything is OK. But before we choose to take the 'ignorance is bliss' route, we owe it to the future to familiarize ourselves with the facts.

I urge everyone to read John Robbin's *Diet for a New America*

(Stillpoint Publishing) and then make a sensible, deliberated decision, based on the truth.

*Spiritual*

If man's ultimate goal is unity, then it is utterly unachievable unless we are prepared to halt exploitation, whether it be to our own kind or beast.

Flesh eating generates materialistic and carnal tendencies, by overstimulating the base chakra (the subtle energy centre at the base of the spine associated with the ego and personal desires and interests) and deadening the senses. It also infiltrates impurity into the consciousness and hinders spiritual growth. By contrast, plant foods are nature's harmonious contributions, possessing subtle qualities that lift and balance. If left untouched after their seasonal maturity, fruit and vegetables would only wither and perish in a relatively short period of time whereas animals' lives are cut short by many years in the process of farming. Thus fruit and vegetables are given to us as gifts of life.

To move forward gracefully, into the new millennium, we must put an end to this needless misery. It's time to do away with cruel and barbaric behaviour and embrace a more compassionate standard. Then in due course we can progress in our spiritual unfoldment, towards personal and planetary peace.

Meat
- is overly high in protein and saturated fat.
- lacks fibre.
- is extremely acid-forming.
- is difficult to digest.
- suppresses the formation of friendly bacteria in the bowel.

Eating factory-farmed animals infiltrates our system with antibiotics, growth and sex hormones and pesticide residues. Being at the top of the food chain, poisons are far more concentrated in animal tissues than in plants. There is also the increased risk of being tarnished with parasites, worms and life-threatening bacterial infections such as *E. coli* and salmonella. And now there's the issue of BSE, which is speculated as being the cause of the fatal Creutzfeldt–Jakob disease (CJD) in humans.

Overconsuming flesh has been directly connected to digestive, liver and kidney disorders, skin troubles, weight gain, diabetes, gallstones, constipation, dullness, fatigue, haemorrhoids, varicose veins, osteoporosis, gout, high blood pressure, clogged arteries, heart disease, colon, breast and prostate cancer and a host of other deep rooted-maladies.

It's quite evident that the human system has not been built to deal with dead  carcasses – hence the numerous conditions that are now correlated with its consumption.

Statistically speaking, evidence reveals that those maintaining a wholefood/vegetarian diet are far less likely to suffer from the typical 'ageing' afflictions of today. They not only have a better quality of life, but live longer too.

Personally, I feel that flesh foods are best excluded from the diet altogether. Except for those who live in extremely cold climates and are limited in the food they can obtain, we do not need the concentrated fat and protein that these items provide. All essential nutrients that we require to stay healthy, can be found abundantly in other domains.

### Seitan

Seitan is an exquisite proteinous meat substitute, made from the gluten in wheat flour. It can be incorporated into stir-fries, casseroles and stews or in any other cooked savoury.

### Tofu

Tofu, or bean curd as it's sometimes termed, is produced from the soya bean and pressed into solid, uniform blocks. Being rather bland, tofu absorbs the flavours of a wide range of ingredients and can replace heavier animal products in both sweet and savoury recipes.

The best way of introducing tofu into the diet is by adding it to simple concoctions such as salads and stir-fries. At first, the smoked and marinated varieties may take away the concern of how to add taste, but with a little practice and experimentation the plain-style slabs can be transformed into irresistible creations.

For idea adaptations, refer to the recipe sections in each season.

### Tempeh

Favoured by the Indonesians, tempeh is a fermented soya bean product that has been meshed together by a special culture called rhizopus. Because it tends to go off rather quickly, it's usually stored in the freezer cabinet and needs to be thawed before use.

Tempeh is highly nutritious, containing almost 20 per cent protein, essential fatty acids and vitamin $B_{12}$, a factor often lacking in the plant world. It also accommodates a natural antibiotic, produced in the fermentation process.

Like tofu, tempeh is easy to work with and can be cooked in a variety of ways. A favourite method is to sauté cubes of it until they are lightly golden, adding a dash of soya sauce or tamari once crisp.

### Fish

Although fish is often extolled by food experts, especially for its omega 3 essential fatty acid content, the main trouble (putting aside the ethical stance) is that most of it is highly contaminated. Swordfish, oysters, mussels and clams definitely contain over-the-limit quantities of toxic metals, and as far as other species are concerned it's hard to know what's safe to eat and what's not. Farmed fish, such as salmon and trout, are also affected by dangerous pesticides.

One thing's for sure, if a fish smells 'fishy' it has already started to rot. I place fish eating in the same league as ingesting other members of the animal kingdom, and for health, moral and spiritual reasons, advise against it.

**Eggs**

Unlike other animal produce, eggs can be considered a 'whole' food rather than a fragmented part and are relatively well assimilated. However, they are certainly not an essential and because they're so condensed, I recommend no more than two a week. If eggs are to be included in the diet, only those from organically raised free-range chickens should be permitted.

**Salt**

Whilst sugar crystals sneak into many of our consumable selections, salt, too, is considerably misused.

Common salt is comprised of two minerals, sodium and chlorine. Although we require both of these tissue salts in our daily diet, more than adequate supplies can be obtained from fresh fruit and vegetables, which also contain plenty of potassium, sodium's synergistic friend.

Although all salt originates from the sea, table salt is mined from the land, where it has long since been deposited. Besides being totally inorganic, it is subjected to a range of supplementary additives including iodine, dextrose (a form of sugar), sodium bicarbonate and usually an aluminium-based anticaking agent to prevent it from clumping.

Sea salt, slightly the lesser of the two evils, possesses on top of its basic make-up small amounts of trace minerals. But beware, most supplies are to some extent still refined. Those that are not are lightly greyish in colour rather than pure white.

Be that as it may, salt intake is generally discouraged, whatever its form. Even after profuse sweating, the electrolytes that are lost through the skin can easily be replenished by drinking a large glass of celery and mixed vegetable juice.

Here are a few good reasons why this crystalline substance is not worth its salt.

Salt
• is acid-forming.

- promotes addiction for more salt and also the need for sugar and alcohol.
- causes a general tissue-salt imbalance.
- An excess intake of salt has been affiliated to water retention, high blood pressure, kidney damage, hardening of the arteries, strokes and heart disease.

The following, although not completely salt-free, can replace commercial salt on the table and in cooking.

### Soya sauce

Fermented from soya beans, wheat, water and sea salt, good quality soya sauce can be used in small quantities. Avoid brands sold in places like supermarkets and grocers as they are usually synthetic and contain sugar, monosodium glutamate, table salt and other cheap offenders. Those brands available from health food stores should contain only pure ingredients.

### Tamari

Tamari is a salty liquid similar to soya sauce, minus the wheat. This makes it suitable for those on a wheat- or gluten-free diet.

### Miso

Miso is a naturally fermented paste produced from cooked soya beans, various grains, sea salt and an organism called koji. It's packed with protein, contains calcium and is also a good source of vitamin $B_{12}$. There are several varieties of miso available, depending on the type of koji employed.

**Hatcho miso** is very dark miso produced from soya bean koji. It's left to ferment for three years and develops a strong, rich flavour. It can be added to soups and casseroles and is particularly appropriate in the winter months.

**Mugi miso** is made from barley koji and is matured for about two years. Mugi is a pleasant, all-year-round choice, and is deeply flavoursome.

**Genmai miso** is fermented from brown rice koji, and like mugi, it takes two years to mature. Being middle of the range, it's not too heavy or overly mild, and can be enjoyed in all kinds of recipes, throughout the year.

**White miso**, or komo miso as it's otherwise known, is produced from white rice and is the mildest and sweetest of misos. It can be incorporated into salad dressings, sauces, pâtés and dips and is more affable in summer.

### Gomasio

Gomasio is a condiment prepared from ground, roasted sesame seeds and sea salt. To make a home-made version, roast 10 heaped tablespoons of sesame seeds in a dry skillet. Then combine it with ½–1 heaped teaspoons of sea salt and blend it in a nut mill. It's great dusted over grains and vegetables or simple sauce-less meals.

### Salt-free zone

#### Celery

Celery's naturally rich sodium content helps provide that saltiness without creating undue imbalance. Chopped fresh celery, celery leaves or the tiny dried seeds can be added to soups and all kinds of savouries.

#### Herbs and spices

Instead of deadening the taste buds with salt, why not experiment with the subtleties of fragrant herbs and gentle spices? Mix and match them sparingly, adding extra if needed, rather than overdoing it first time round. Use fresh herbs in the spring and summer, resorting to the dried or hardier versions when it's cold. For further information on culinary herbs, turn to page 95.

*Bragg's Liquid Aminos*

This is a delightful vegetable protein seasoning, similar to tamari and soya sauce. Rich in 16 amino acids, unlike the latter it's unfermented and contains no added salt.

*Seaweed*

Having come from the ocean, sea vegetables are ideal salt replacers, highly endowed with a mixture of minerals and other added extras. Toasted nori flakes and roasted ground dulse are particularly satisfying, and can be sprinkled over grains, beans, vegetables and anything else fanciable.

# CHAPTER 4

# Diet and Climate

We've touched on how different foods affect our health, both positively and negatively. Keeping this in mind, we can now move on and begin to link the basic dietary principles to climate and location.

On the whole, the type of food we eat should largely depend on where we reside and the produce that grows there. In warm climates there tends to be an abundance of light and cooling crops, whereas food growing in colder regions is of a much heartier quality.[1] Through this simple complementary system, nature never fails to keep us in balance.

Eating fruit and vegetables that grow in our vicinity is especially important, as being seasonal they are closely linked to the essence of the land. Even if they do not originate in the country in which they are being successfully grown (for example, potatoes and tomatoes originally come from South America but grow well in many parts of Europe), the fact that they are able to grow healthily suggests that they are suitable crops for that environment and the people who live there. However, for the sake of practicality, grains, legumes, seeds, nuts and seaweed may be transported from one country to another, providing they have been exposed to similar atmospheric conditions and are situated on the same side of the equator.

While the exchange of produce from East to West is not ideal, it's acceptable as it does not oppose the seasonal flow (the seasons experienced are the same). However, food that is carried from one side of the equator to the other, due to the housing of opposite influences (the seasons are experienced the opposite) may subtly affect our health. For this reason, the trade of Northern- and Southern-hemisphere crops is best avoided.

If we choose to move from one location to another, whether it be short or long term, it's important that we observe the eating habits of our new environment and adjust our diet to suit it.

To portray the value of eating what grows around us, here are five good reasons why local food is best.

- Eating local crops helps us adapt to our environment, keeping us in tune with climate and season.
- Locally grown foodstuff is fresher (it hasn't been transported for thousands of miles), so therefore contains more nutrients. Some vegetables can lose up to 50 per cent of their vitamin C content within two or three days – so the quicker they get to us, the better.
- Living off local produce helps strengthen our immunity, making us less prone to local disease. This is achieved by the harmonizing of our blood and inner body chemistry with our outer surroundings.
- Imported foods are likely to require more chemicals to keep them fresh, so that they last longer. Some of these toxins may be illegal in our own country, but because this information does not need to be provided, we'll never know.
- Home-grown food reduces pollution output, by cutting the need for extensive transportation. Consequently, this will decrease the effect of global warming.

To give an example of the intimate link between food and climate, I shall briefly recall a short story.

About 30 years ago, a friend's father came from India to live in England. Being familiar with his traditional diet of hot, fiery food, he continued to eat his indigenous Indian fare. However, it wasn't long after that he started to develop severe digestive problems and his health deteriorated. Yet whenever he returned to his homeland for holidays, he noticed his symptoms miraculously disappeared. Realizing his suffering was somehow associated with what he ate and where he ate it, he tried miserably to change his diet. Failing to make the necessary transition, he decided to return to India permanently, where he has maintained good health ever since.

## THE CLIMATE ZONES

To help classify climatic consumption, we can divide the globe into five regions: polar, cool, temperate, semi-tropical and tropical.

### Polar dietary zone

The polar areas include the countries that lie nearest to the poles, such as Greenland in the north. The few inhabited islands that exist here have predominantly cold weather extremes throughout the year. People living in these regions require plenty of warmth, obtainable from a more consolidated, cooked regime. A large proportion of the diet (up to 80 per cent) should be made up of wholegrains such as buckwheat, oats, winter millet and wheat. These grains are the most heat-producing of all cereals and thrive in cooler climates. Vegetables are mainly of the root and sea varieties and require relatively long cooking times. Legumes, nuts and seeds, together with eggs and if necessary fish, can also be moderately incorporated, particularly when temperatures are very low. Animal produce should be traditionally prepared and be free from commercial farming hazards.

### Cool dietary zone

In cool districts of the world, such as Scandinavia and Alaska, we see climatic conditions that generally exhibit long winters and short summers. Similarly to polar areas, dietary needs revolve around plenty of grain: buckwheat, millet, short grain brown rice, wheat, barley and oats, together with smaller amounts of legumes, seeds and nuts. Land and sea vegetables should be for the most part cooked, with the addition of some raw, seasonal fruit and vegetables introduced in the warmer months. Eggs and small quantities of goat's milk produce can also be taken.

## Temperate dietary zone

In regions such as Europe and most of North America, the climate is known as a temperate one, and has four distinct seasons. Rather than staying with the same kind of dietary pattern all year round, meals must be adjusted to each seasonal swing as external changes occur.

In the spring and summer months, the diet should consist of approximately 25–35 per cent grains, combined with some legumes, seeds, nuts, plenty of sprouted grains and raw fruit and vegetables. When cooking, the lighter methods such as stir-frying and steaming are preferable, so that the food still remains crisp and fresh.

As autumn and winter begin to set in, entertain larger quantities of cereals and slightly more beans. Vegetables can be cooked using longer softening techniques; except for the dried varieties, fruit should be minimal. Simmering seasonal fruit in a little juice is another way of taking off the cooling edge to this food group. Eggs and goat's milk produce may be taken occasionally if desired.

## Semi-tropical dietary zone

People living in semi-tropical zones, as we witness in Northern Australia and South America, experience the opposite of cool-climate locations, with long hot summers and comparatively short, mild winters. Those residing in such regions require a much lighter, alkaline-forming diet, with less cooked food and plenty of fruit and raw leafy and flowering vegetables. Medium- to long-grain brown rice and other less compact grains are the cereals of choice, together with small quantities of beans, seeds and nuts. Due to its richness, animal produce should be limited or avoided.

**Tropical dietary zone**

In tropical parts of the world, such as India, South-East Asia and the central strip of Africa, the land is exposed to high temperatures all year through. Such a climate gives rise to an abundance of tropical fruits, seeds and nuts and an array of indigenous vegetables. Besides fruit, most plants are eaten cooked in the tropics, as raw foods are likely to harbour dangerous microorganisms which are killed in the cooking process.

Grains include rice, barley, corn and other cereals, which are commonly eaten with spicy vegetable sauces. Many spices, although initially warming, ultimately produce heat loss.

As in sub-tropical countries, those living in the tropics do not require animal produce. Ideally, a vegan lifestyle is the one of choice here.

# CHAPTER 5

# An Introduction to the Seasons

At last, we've made it. We've ventured through the good, the bad and the ugly and now we can finally cross the border, into the main theme of the book – living and eating with the seasons.

Although the information is based on zones that experience a four-season cycle, it can easily be adapted to other climatic locations by referring to the relevant pages. For example, the weather in Mexico (semi-tropical zone) remains fairly hot most of the year, with only a very short mild spell. People living in this realm will therefore, on the whole, need to refer to the guidelines set out in the chapters on spring and summer. Those who reside in countries that are prone to extreme weather conditions, eg tropic or polar regions, should link up with the season that most resembles their particular climate. Traditional crops, which may not all be mentioned in the food guides, can also be incorporated here.

Please note that the fresh fruit and vegetables included in the seasonal shopping guides are in accord with the temperate zones in the Northern hemisphere. As the timing of produce in temperate zones may vary from country to country, some crops may not be available until the latter part of the season.

For simplicity, the four seasons are covered individually, with a chapter for each one. At the end of each chapter there's a special guide to what's in season and a chance to put theory into practice with a selection of tried and tested recipes.

**Recipes and eating with the seasons**

The recipes in this book are largely vegan, although the occasional inclusion of free-range eggs and vegetarian goat's cheese has been permitted. Those following a vegan diet can for the most part replace these products with soya cheese and egg replacer. Sugar and all refined products have been strictly banned and the addition of sea salt is optional (turn to page 33 for healthy alternatives).

When you don the chef's hat and apron strings and cook up a seasonal surprise, remember the kitchen recommendations:

- Wherever possible, purchase organic produce.
- Filter all water before use.
- Choose only unrefined vegetable oils.
- Wash legumes, grains, vegetables and fruit well.

## THE FOUR SEASONS

Before we set foot on this wondrous expedition, let's sit back and take a few minutes to reflect on the diverse scenarios of the year.

> The hedge, once black like twisted iron, is now enlaced with tender leaves
> Green of budding honeysuckle foams about the cottage eaves . . .
> In the orchard overnight, a mist has come: a rosy haze –
> where the swelling apple bloom is breaking on the clustered sprays.

* * *

> The wheat is like a sun-flecked sea beneath the summer sky –
> little ripples break the surface as the wind slips by . . .
> Here and there the scarlet poppies with their petals wide
> rise and dip like red-sailed vessels on the rolling tide.

\* \* \*

Drifting mist and burning colour – all along the garden ways . . .
Blue smoke rising from the chimneys through the soft and silvery
  haze.
Webs upon the spangled hedges. Wisps of gauze upon the lawn . . .
Autumn roses, pink and golden,
in the grey October dawn.

\* \* \*

The crunch of ice beneath your tread.
The leafless branches overhead.
A wayside cottage thatched with snow . . .
The hedge with hips and haws aglow
becomes a strange and lovely sight
in the bright and frosty light.
Along the lanes you know so well
beauty casts a magic spell.
There's so much to see and much to learn.
At every gate and every turn
you see what summer's green concealed;
the distant spire, the far-off field.
For when the trees stand stripped and bare
they open windows everywhere . . .
A different landscape you survey
walking on a winter's day.

PATIENCE STRONG,
'Through the Year'

Each season has something to offer. In approximately 365 days we witness the birth (spring), growth (summer), maturity (autumn) and death (winter) of the land, only for it to be reborn again the following year. Our own lives, too, mirror this same unending cycle, spread out throughout our lifetime. And for those of us who believe in the dance of reincarnation, death, like the winter, is but a mere rest.

If we have an abhorrence or a liking for one season over all others, then very often it can reveal an imbalance. The ancient

Chinese law of the Five Elements associates each season with different organs of the body. Therefore a personal link to a particular time of year could mean a problem with interacting organs. For example, an aversion to or favouring of autumn might suggest a weakness in the area of the lungs and/or large intestine.

*Figure 8, The season–organ associations in accordance with the Law of the Five Elements[1]*

| Season | Element | Organs |
| --- | --- | --- |
| spring | wood | liver and gall bladder |
| summer | fire | heart and small intestine |
| late summer | earth | spleen and stomach |
| autumn | metal | lungs and large intestine |
| winter | water | kidneys and bladder |

An instability with any of the seasons can usually be resolved by choosing to live alongside nature rather than against her. This can be accomplished by pursuing the *Eating with the Seasons* principles and listening to one's inner voice.

For those who feel they may be in need of a little assistance, a course of Five-Element acupuncture, performed by an experienced practitioner, can help retune the body with the elements, restoring an affinity between one's inner self and the environment.

Let's now enter the first season of the year and explore the charms of spring.

# CHAPTER 6

# Spring

*When the hounds of Spring are on Winter's traces,*
*The mother of months in meadow or plain*
*Fills the shadows and windy places*
*With lisp of leaves and ripple of rain.*

ALGERNON CHARLES SWINBURNE

Spring is officially delivered on 20 March,[1] at the time when the sun crosses the equator and day equals night. This balancing act is known as the spring equinox.

If we look around us at this time of year, we can see nature awaking from her winter slumber, ready to make a fresh start. Like a biological clock, spring gives birth to a budding creation, bringing newness and hope to all that it touches.

For us too it's a season of renewal and regeneration. It's a time to shake off the old and embrace the new. We may wish to try out new ventures, meet new people and begin to sow the seeds of our winter dreams. It also provides us with a second chance to rekindle our new year's resolutions and make another go of things.

During the spring, we should gradually require less sleep and be able to get up a little earlier. Rising with the morning light is an ideal time to awake. As darkness meets dawn, yin and yang become one, engaging in a harmonious treaty.

We can make the most of the extra time by doing something meaningful – whether it be meditation, yoga or a more physically active pursuit. Giving ourselves some space before the hustle and bustle of the day sets in can change how we deal with forthcoming situations, and improve the quality of our life no end. Just 10 to 15 minutes of quiet can make all the difference.

# A SPRING DIET

As spring comes out of its shell, we can start to think about changing our choice of diet from a weightier winter one to a slightly lighter mix. This shift can be made over a period of several weeks, as early spring in many places is still rather cool.

The best way of making the transition is to eat a little less cooked food and a little more raw. There should be no difficulty in doing this as nature produces an array of crisp spring vegetables, in perfect synchronicity with our body's needs. Broccoli, new spring roots (baby carrots, turnips and spring onions) and an assortment of dark leafy greens are just some of the seasonal contenders. Sprouted foods also make an appropriate addition.

Fresh herbs out and about at this time of year include mint and parsley, two flavoursome favourites. Sprinkle chopped mint on to new potatoes and carrots or steep up a bunch in a saucepan of boiling water to perfect some home-brewed mint tea. Parsley, a herb that works well as a water-retention reliever, can also be brewed into a therapeutic infusion or used in almost any dish. Parsley is a top source of antioxidants, containing three times as much vitamin C as oranges, and nibbled on after indulging in anything fried can deactivate potential toxicity.

With fruit still quite limited in temperate parts of the globe in spring, the amount we eat must be restricted too. Avoid purchasing tropical or Southern hemisphere produce, as it will only cause imbalance. Stay with locally grown offerings; one or two pieces a day are sufficient.

### Go green

Kale, spinach, watercress and mustard greens are a few of the nutritious leaves that befall us in the spring. Rich in beta carotene, folic acid (important prior to and during pregnancy), vitamin C, calcium and iron, these greens contain the wealthiest concentration of minerals of all other land plants. They are also low in fat, high in fibre and possess one of nature's most powerful healers – chlorophyll.

Chlorophyll is the green pigment present in plants and functions to convert light energy from the sun into more tangible substances. Although chlorophyll is found in all plant life, the greener the plant the more chlorophyll it contains. Dark, leafy greens are therefore a particularly good source.

Eating foods that are rich in this component has been shown to exert a range of beneficial actions, including oxygenating the body and boosting the red blood cell count. This is probably linked to the fact that chlorophyll has similar characteristics to that of haemoglobin, the red pigment in blood.

Chlorophyll also promotes the growth of the good intestinal flora, inhibits the multiplication of cancer cells and helps eliminate unpleasant body odours. That's why chewing a sprig of parsley after eating garlic or onions arrests the smell.

A further effect of chlorophyll is its ability to detoxify. It's an excellent agent for clearing waste materials from the blood and liver and is a vital element to include during a spring cleanse.

To become familiar with some of spring's chlorophyll-packed veg, try adding them to soups, stir-fries and salads or combine them with other vegetables and put them through a juicer. Why not go ahead and give some of the following greens the green light?

- beet greens
- cabbage
- collard greens
- dandelion greens
- kale
- mustard greens
- spinach
- Swiss chard
- turnip greens
- watercress

Some greens contain significant amounts of oxalic acid and need to be lightly cooked to neutralize this substance. For further information concerning naturally occurring oxalic acid, turn back to page 17.

## Super sprouts

Another food group that's only been skimmed over so far is sprouts. By this I'm not referring to the Brussels variety most of us eat at Christmas, but to dried seeds that when germinated grow into mouthwatering salad.

Sprouts are perfect for the spring. They bridge the gap between March's modest platter and July's raw food extravagance. Sprouting also provides us with another way of enjoying grains and legumes, which would otherwise be inedible if left uncooked.

Dry seeds (in this case, when I signify seeds, I'm referring to anything that will sprout, which includes legumes and grains as well) are a storehouse of nourishment. When we sprout them, through the process of photosynthesis (the combination of water, oxygen and light) their locked-in nutrition is unleashed, leaving us with crunchy, power-packed plants.

The miracle of germination causes several changes to occur to a seed:

- Nutrients are broken down into more easily digestible compounds: proteins into amino acids, starches into simple carbohydrates and fats into essential fatty acids.
- Vitamin and mineral content is increased by between 200 and 2,000 per cent.
- Minerals are more freely absorbed, due to improved chelation.
- Enzymes are produced, aiding food assimilation.
- Chlorophyll is manufactured.
- Calories are reduced.
- Water content rises.
- The gluten in sprouted wheat virtually disappears.
- Toxins that are present in some legumes which inhibit protein digestion are eliminated.
- Canavanin, a toxin found in alfalfa seeds, is nullified.

- The energy of the seed is changed from a warming vibration to a cooling one – ideal for spring. For an understanding of the warming and cooling potential of different foods, please refer to page 161.
- Sprouts are cost-efficient – 1 tablespoon of dry seed is equivalent to approximately 8 tablespoons of sprouts.

Sprouts can be said to be 'live' food. This is because if we eat them at the right stage of germination, their energy is still very active. Although the life force in fully grown vegetables is strong as well, the vitality in a sprout is far superior.

Whilst a limited selection of sprouts can be purchased ready-to-eat, it's far better to grow them at home. Germinating sprouts is fun to do, requiring no soil or fertilizer. All that is needed is some seeds, an apparatus to grow them in, filtered water and a little care. Here are five simple steps to creating an indoor sprout garden. Before commencing, either purchase a commercial sprouter from a local health-food store or acquire a wicker basket, a plastic colander, a sieve or a flower pot.

*Figure 9, Sprouting seeds and their harvest time. Beginners should start by sprouting those seeds listed in the left-hand column. These varieties are easy to produce and need minimum attention. Once they have been mastered, those in the right-hand column can be put to the test.*[2]

| Seed | Harvest time in days | Seed | Harvest time in days |
|------|----------------------|------|----------------------|
| alfalfa | 5–7 | barley | 3–4 |
| adzuki beans | 4–6 | black-eyed beans | 3–5 |
| chickpeas | 4 | buckwheat | 4–5 |
| fenugreek | 4–5 | flageolet beans | 3–5 |
| green lentils | 3–5 | haricot beans | 3–5 |
| mung beans | 2–3 | millet | 2–3 |
| radish seeds | 4–5 | oats | 2–3 |
| soya beans | 3–6 | peas | 3–5 |
| wheat | 2–4 | pumpkin seeds | 2–4 |
| | | rice | 2–3 |
| | | rye | 3–5 |
| | | sesame seeds | 3–4 |
| | | sunflower seeds | 4–5 |

1 Soak the seeds of choice overnight in plenty of water.
2 Drain and rinse the seeds well and place a thin layer of them in the base of the sprouter. If the holes in the bottom of the sprouter are too large, line it with a sheet of muslin or cheese-cloth, to prevent the seeds from falling through.
3 Leave the sprouter in the kitchen, away from direct sunlight.
4 Rinse the seeds two to three times a day, for about 30 seconds at a time. This helps wash away debris given off by the chemical processes during germination and provides the sprouts with a fresh supply of water. Always drain them well or they can begin to rot. But do not allow them to dry out.
5 Continue to rinse until ready to harvest. See figure 9 for correct gathering times. Then give them one final wash, remove them from the sprouter and store them in the fridge. Mature sprouts are best eaten within one week.

**Spring cooking techniques**

As we move from the colder part of the calendar to a warmer one, it's not just our choice of food that will differ but how we prepare and cook it as well.

Adapting our cooking techniques to the spring requires openness and flexibility, as we're likely to come up against an assortment of weather conditions. In some regions, spring bursts forth full-on and we'll automatically feel a need for dietary change. In other areas, spring may take time to settle. On these unpredictable days, it's best not to venture too far from a winter regime. But as the environment starts to warm up, we can begin to cook and eat lighter, in preparation for the sunshine months ahead.

*Steaming and waterless cooking*

Sensible cooking practices for this time of year include methods that are quick and use minimal heat. Steaming is the most reliable way of softening vegetables, as they don't come into direct contact with the cooking water, resulting in less nutrient loss and firmer food.

Waterless cooking, where the vegetables are left to simmer in their own juices, is also serviceable. For this technique, thick bottomed stainless steel saucepans or special waterless cookware are a worthwhile investment.

## Stir-frying

Stir-frying is another excellent way of cooking spring edibles. The flavours and nutrients from a variety of foods can be combined to form satisfying, easy-to-prepare meals. Use a tablespoonful of oil at the most (olive, peanut or sesame), adding water or stock if the pan gets too dry. Take care not to overcook. Stir-fried meals shouldn't turn out soggy.

## Blanching

Although boiling vegetables is not really the done thing, there are one or two exceptions to the rule. Quick boiling (immersing food into boiling water for a matter of minutes), or blanching as it's otherwise known, is one way of eliminating complete rawness without interfering too much with nutrient content. Cauliflower and broccoli turn out well with this method, especially when used for their role in salads. Steaming these members of the Cruciferae family may destroy some of the cancer-fighting substances typically found in this class of food.

Dark leafy greens are also suited to the quick boil, as much of the oxalic acid found in some varieties is eliminated. Even if partial leaching of nutrients occurs, greens are so richly endowed there will always be substantial amounts left behind.

## Boiling

Whilst immersing vegetables in a pan full of boiling water is the last method of choice when cooking this food group, grains and beans boil up exceptionally well. Dried foods need to absorb sufficient water for the softening process, making this technique ideal. When cooking grains, it's best to follow the instructions on the packet, so they don't turn out mushy or undercooked. With legumes, as long as the pan doesn't dry out being precise about how much liquid to use is not as important.

*Raw food*

Uncooked foods also play an important role in the spring transition, and salads and sprouts should be an everyday feature. For a seasonal salad informer, turn to the spring shopping guide on page 75 or try out some of the raw recipe recommendations at the end of this chapter.

## SPRING CLEANSING

There's no better time to commit to an inner cleanse than at the beginning of this season. As the spring equinox dawns, the energy of the land is fully geared into elimination. Even if we don't make an effort to work with it, toxins will be drawn out of the body, sometimes causing us to feel quite unwell. But if we go with the flow and submit ourselves to nature's doings, the benefits will be assured.

Embarking on a cleanse doesn't have to be anything too drastic – it can be as easygoing or as disciplined as we want to make it. Before commencing, it's always wise to ascertain that the bowel is functioning regularly, at least once or twice a day. This is to ensure that the toxins that are thrown out of the blood and liver are carried efficiently away. If the lower alimentary canal isn't working as well as it should be, poisons can be reabsorbed into the system, or make their way out via other exits, as is often seen in a spotty skin.

To ensure optimum bowel movements, the following intestinal aids can be supplemented two weeks before and during the cleanse.

*Psyllium husks*

A powdered soluble fibre that absorbs toxins, increases bowel transit time (the length of time it takes for food to travel through the system) and provides intestinal bulk. Begin on a low dose, one heaped teaspoon twice a day, together with a large glass of water. As the body becomes more adjusted to the increased amount of fibre, the dosage can be gradually upped. A sufficient volume of fluid must always be consumed when taking psyllium husks, so as to impart a medium where it can properly expand.

*Linseeds*

Besides being an excellent source of essential fatty acids, these small, oily seeds function as an intestinal lubricant. Take one heaped dessertspoonful morning and evening with a glass of water.

*Aloe vera juice*

The juice from the leaves of the aloe vera plant comprises a multitude of outstanding substances, many of which have the ability to cleanse and soothe the entire alimentary canal. It also helps provide a healthy environment for the friendly intestinal bacteria to flourish. As the concentration of aloe vera juice varies from brand to brand, the dosage followed should be in accordance with the manufacturer's directions.

**Seven-day spring clean-out programme**

A procedure I have followed every spring for the last few years is a simple seven-day clean-out routine, based around grains and vegetables. Some seasonal fruit and freshly squeezed fruit juices are also included, but as these can sometimes be overly eliminative sticking to them for just a day or so in the middle of the programme is ample.

Several days before starting out on the programme, all animal and dairy produce, sugar, wheat, processed and refined foods, tea, coffee and alcohol must be eliminated. For those who are used to allowing these substances in their diet, this elimination period may be conducted over several weeks. A juicer will be very useful.

For information on what fruit and vegetables to include in the cleanse, refer to the spring shopping guide on page 75. More information on juices can be found on page 92, in the Summer section.

Having established a regular wholefood eating pattern the clean-out programme can be commenced.

The cleansing routine set out is not over-the-top, allowing most of us to attempt it without too much trouble. And apart from having to kit our kitchens out with the required preparations, we can carry on with our normal daytime drill.

Throughout the cleanse, it's vital to drink plenty of water between meals. On day 5 of the programme, where liquid only is taken, water can be drunk at any time. Vegetable juices and herb teas can also be included throughout all of the seven days (nettle is good). Fresh vegetable juices are one of the most healing gifts we can feed our bodies. They are rich in antioxidants and enzymes, which are released instantly into the bloodstream, without having to be digested. They also possess large quantities of magnesium and potassium, two minerals that alkalize the blood and help to remove toxins from inside the cells.

*Days 1 and 2*

Eat organic short-grain brown rice and steamed vegetables.

It's important to begin the cleanse by consuming grains and steamed vegetables on the first two days, to allow the body to become accustomed to a heightened elimination. Brown rice and softened vegetables are gentle cleaners, the fibres in the cereals helping to absorb toxins from the colon. The rice and vegetables can be eaten as three main meals, or four or five smaller meals.

### Day 3

Eat organic short-grain brown rice and raw vegetables.

Eat the grains and vegetables as three main meals or four or five smaller ones as before.

### Day 4

Eat raw vegetables and seasonal fruit only.

As the detoxification progresses, raw food, which has a stronger cleansing impact, can be introduced. As much fruit and vegetables can be taken as desired, although the two food groups are best not consumed at the same time.

### Day 5

Drink raw vegetable and fruit juices only. Include no solids.

Having access to a juicer is an essential requirement here, although shop-bought freshly pressed products can be supplemented. Always try to buy organic produce, as juices, being highly concentrated, are likely to be concentrated in pesticides. This juice-only day can be extended if wished, but if you've never fasted before, please OK it with a GP or dietary therapist beforehand.

### Days 6 and 7

Eat organic short-grain brown rice and steamed vegetables.

### After the clean-out

It's important to reintroduce other foods slowly, so as not to overburden the system. This can be done over several days. Acidophilus and bifido, two strains of 'friendly' bacteria that populate the colon, are often washed away during a cleanse and must be replenished. Powdered or encapsulated products can be purchased from most health food stores and require taking twice a day on an empty stomach. The administration of aloe vera juice can also be maintained.

To conserve the health and cleanliness of the system, a one-day-a-week or fortnightly juice fast can be continued through the spring and summer.

It's not just our bodies that require a rinse in the spring, but our living quarters too. Over the weeks, months and years, we tend to accumulate unnecessary hotchpotch. We hold on to things we don't really need. According to Feng Shui, the ancient art of placement, this can block the energy flow in the rooms of our home, which may sooner or later impede various aspects of our life.

On a quiet weekend, spend some time having a really thorough spruce. Clear out cluttered cupboards, dusty drawers and weighed-down wardrobes. Donate no longer needed clothes, ornaments and bric-à-brac to a local charity shop and throw away anything that's past its sell-by date.

Following this revamp, don't be surprised at the many positive changes that are likely to appear.

**Balanced weight**

Spring is frequently a time when many of us wish to shed a few pounds, often put on throughout the winter. Balancing our weight is fundamentally all about balancing what we eat. We don't have to engage ourselves in fad dieting systems or drastically restrict calories to reach our goal (although a rough count won't go amiss). In fact these types of reducing attempts actually cause our metabolic rate to slow down, which motivates the body to hang on tightly to every ounce.

By following the seasonal eating guidelines set out in this book, an achievable weight can be guaranteed.

To help shift the excess baggage, a spring cleanse like the one set out on pages 68–70, is a good place to start. This common custom guarantees to clear away rubbish, promote fat loss and give the digestive system a bit of a much needed rest.

Once the detox is through, here are some fat-conquering suggestions to follow.

- Always drink plenty of water in between meals to ease hunger. Keeping the body well hydrated is the most effective means of stabilizing the blood-sugar level, preventing cravings and fatigue. Do not take liquids with meals, as it can interfere with food breakdown, by diluting digestive enzymes.
- Keep well away from fried food and all saturated and hydrogenated fats.
- Stick to high-fibre eating. Include a large plate of vegetables (raw or cooked) at both midday and evening meals.
- If animal produce is included in the diet, make sure that protein and starchy foods are eaten at least four hours apart from each other. This aids digestibility and assimilation of meals. For more details see the food-combining section on page 100 and read *Food Combining for Health* by Doris Grant and Jean Joice and *Food Combining for Vegetarians* by Jackie Le Tissier.
- Try not to eat after the sun goes down, when the digestive process is at its weakest. In the winter, this can mean eating the last meal rather early. An option here is to eat a slightly heavier meal at midday (this is the ideal) and just munch on fruit or vegetables or drink a light soup in the evening. Eating two to three hours before retiring, whatever the season, should be prohibited.
- Don't skip meals in the hope of losing extra weight. This only slows down the metabolic rate, making weight loss even harder.
- Only eat when hungry. Very often it's our thirst that needs quenching and not the stomach that needs filling.
- Exclude personal allergy-producing foods, as they can trigger bloating and weight gain.
- Shun food shopping when you're hungry. Temptation time will loom large and resistance may prove to be difficult.
- Never eat when stressed or emotionally upset, as digestive enzymes fail to function properly. Try pacification through

other means, such as taking a warm bath, talking to a friend or going for a walk or a jog.

- Let go of fear. On a deeper level, having a few too many layers can indicate a subconscious attempt to protect ourselves. The Australian Bush flower remedies Dog Rose or Grey Spider Flower may help release this crippling emotion.

- Attend a local sports hall or health club at least three times a week and get physically fit. Vary exercise to include aerobic, toning and weight-bearing activity. Research shows that the more muscle we have, the faster we burn fat. Ask a fitness instructor to work out a personal exercise plan.

- If snacking is an occasional (or regular) must, exchange high fat/sugar munchies for some of these less guilt-laden treats: fresh or dried fruit, rice cakes with tahini or sugar-free jam, rice crackers, plain popcorn, crudités with low fat humus and soya yoghurt. Also hunt through the confectionery section in local health food stores to find a hoard of innocent delicacies.

Here are five aids to help expedite a slim, trim physique. They can enhance fat loss when combined with a sensible wholefood diet, sufficient filtered water and a regular exercise regime.

*Flaxseed oil*

Flaxseed oil contains the essential fats the body needs. Studies suggest that these 'good' fats regulate the action of insulin, helping us to use carbohydrates and fats for fuel more efficiently.
Dose: 1tbsp (UK)/1½tbsp (US) daily.

*Spirulina*

Spirulina is a rich source of vitamins, minerals, amino acids and enzymes. It enhances metabolism, and taken before meals suppresses the appetite.
Dose: Up to 3000mg one hour before main meals.

*L. carnitine*

The amino acid *L. carnitine* carries stored fat to muscle cells, where it's easier to use as fuel.
Dose: 500–1000mg on an empty stomach morning and evening.

*Chromium picolinate*

Chromium helps the body to increase muscle growth and utilize fat. It also aids the stabilization of blood glucose, easing cravings for sugar and stimulants.
Dose: One 200–500mcg capsule daily, after food.

*Lipotropic factors*

The amino acid methionine together with choline and inositol are what is known as lipotropic factors. By increasing the production of lecithin in the liver, these nutrients function to keep lipids and cholesterol more soluble, thereby making fat easier for the body to manoeuvre. They also help to maintain liver health.
Dose: one tablet or capsule after each meal.

## SPRING REVIEW

1. Eat more raw foods and fewer cooked.
2. Embark on a spring cleanse.
3. Clear out the living quarters.
4. Get juicing and start germinating sprouts.
5. Lose excess weight.
6. Start an exercise schedule, if one is not already in practice.
7. Do away with eating habits that don't support good health.

To conclude our visit to spring, here's a shopping guide to the fresh produce in season. It also includes a variety of dried wholefoods, which although aren't distinctive of spring are essential store-cupboard provisions.

*Figure 10, Fresh foods in spring*

| Vegetables | Herbs | Grains | Beans/Pulses |
|---|---|---|---|
| asparagus | basil | amaranth | adzuki |
| beetroot | bay leaf | barley | black turtle |
| broccoli | chives | buckwheat | black-eyed |
| cabbage | coriander leaf | bulgar wheat | borlotti |
| carrots | dandelion | maize | broad |
| cauliflower | dill | millet | cannellini |
| celery | marjoram | oats | chickpeas |
| chicory | mint | quinoa | field |
| Chinese leaves | nettle | rice | flageolet |
| courgettes or | oregano | wheat | haricot |
|    zucchini | parsley | wild rice | lentils |
| cress | rosemary | | mung |
| globe artichokes | sage | | pinto |
| greens | sorrel | | red kidney |
| kale | tarragon | | soya |
| leeks | thyme | | split peas |
| mushrooms | | | |
| onions | | | |
| parsnips | | | |
| peas | | | |
| potatoes | | | |
| radish | | | |
| spinach | | | |
| Swiss chard | | | |
| turnips | | | |
| watercress | | | |

| Sprouts | Seeds | Nuts | Fruit |
|---|---|---|---|
| All sprouted | hemp | almonds | apples |
|    grains, legumes | linseed | Brazils | dried fruit |
|    and seeds | pumkin | cashews | pears |
| | sesame | chestnuts | rhubarb |
| | sunflower | hazelnuts | |
| | | macadamias | |
| | | peanuts | |
| | | pecans | |
| | | pine nuts | |
| | | pistachios | |
| | | walnuts | |

# RECIPES FOR SPRING

## Mixed Bean and Spring Onion Salad
*Serves 8*

INGREDIENTS
225g/8oz red kidney beans, soaked overnight
225g/8oz chickpeas, soaked overnight
1 strip of kombu, rehydrated
100g/4oz sprouted mung beans
25g/1oz sun-dried tomatoes, soaked in boiling water for 30 minutes
170g/6oz celery, finely chopped
3 spring onions, trimmed and finely chopped
One 100g/4oz box of mustard and cress, trimmed
Dressing
1 heaped tbsp freeze-dried tarragon
1tbsp (UK)/1½tbsp (US) safflower oil
1tbsp (UK)/1½tbsp (US) cider vinegar
2tsp (UK)/2tsp (US) whole-grain mustard

Drain the legumes and rinse well. Place them in a saucepan of boiling water together with the kombu and simmer for 2 hours until soft. Drain and place in a bowl.

Add the other ingredients and the dressing ingredients and mix.

## New Potato Salad with Horseradish and Mint
*Serves 6*

INGREDIENTS
200g/7oz red kidney beans, soaked overnight
1 strip of kombu, rehydrated
900g/2lb new potatoes
200g/7oz mangetout, trimmed
200g/7oz radish, trimmed and finely sliced
4 spring onions, trimmed and chopped
Dressing
3 heaped tbsp chopped fresh parsley
2 heaped tsp finely grated wild horseradish
2 heaped tsp chopped fresh mint
4tbsp (UK)/⅓C(US) tofu mayonnaise (available from health-food stores)
sea salt

Drain and rinse the beans and simmer in boiling water with the kombu for 2 hours or until soft. Drain and set aside.

Halve the new potatoes and steam with the mangetout for 10–15 minutes. Place the cooked beans, potatoes and mangetout in a bowl and add the radish and spring onion. Combine the dressing ingredients, and mix into the salad.

## Japanese Sprouted Wheat Salad
*Serves 6–8*

INGREDIENTS
25g/1oz hijiki, soaked for 15 minutes in water
200g/7oz sprouted wheat
100g/4oz spring greens, finely sliced
100g/4oz radish, trimmed and finely sliced
2 heaped tbsp gomasio
Dressing
2tbsp (UK)/3tbsp(US) sesame oil
1tbsp (UK)/1½tbsp (US) brown rice vinegar
1tsp (UK)/1tsp (US) soya sauce or tamari

Drain the excess liquid from the hijiki and steam or simmer for 45 minutes until soft. Place it in a bowl, add the sprouted wheat, spring greens, radish and gomasio and combine. Mix the dressing ingredients together and stir into the salad.


## Mixed Leaf Salad with Feta Cheese and Artichoke Dressing
*Serves 6*

INGREDIENTS
250g/9oz mixed lettuce, eg curly endive, radicchio, lollo rosso, iceberg
2 heaped tbsp finely chopped chives
100g/4oz vegetarian feta cheese, cubed
Dressing
400g/14oz can of artichoke hearts, drained
2tbsp (UK)/3tbsp(US) sunflower oil
1tbsp (UK)/1½tbsp (US) lemon juice
Half a clove of garlic, crushed
1 heaped tsp mild chilli powder
125ml/4½fl oz (UK)/½C (US) carrot or mixed vegetable juice
sea salt

Place the lettuce leaves, chives and feta cheese in a bowl and mix. Blend the dressing ingredients together in a liquidizer until smooth, chill and serve with the salad.

**Greek Pasta Salad**
*Serves 6*

INGREDIENTS
300g/11oz wholewheat, spelt or rice pasta swirls
3 tomatoes, chopped
Half a medium cucumber, peeled and diced
1 spring onion, chopped
100g/4oz pickled gherkins, chopped
100g/4oz black French olives
50g/2oz vegetarian feta cheese or firm soya cheese, cubed
5 heaped tbsp finely chopped fresh parsley
3 tbsp (UK)/¼C (US) olive oil
sea salt and black pepper

Boil the pasta according to the instructions on the packet, drain and place in a bowl. Add the tomatoes, cucumber, spring onion, pickled gherkins, olives, cheese, parsley, olive oil, salt and pepper and mix.

**Brown Rice with Seitan and Vegetables**
*Serves 4*

INGREDIENTS
350g/12oz brown rice
250g/9oz leeks, trimmed and chopped
250g/9oz carrots, peeled and cut into thin small sticks
200g/7oz seitan, cut into medium-sized pieces
3 tbsp (UK)/¼C (US) sesame oil
1 small cauliflower, trimmed and cut into florets
300ml/10fl oz (UK)/1¼C (US) water
2 heaped tsp miso
2 heaped tbsp grated ginger root
1 heaped tbsp tamari
2 heaped tsp kuzu root

Simmer the rice in twice the volume of water (or more if necessary) for 30 minutes and set aside. Sauté the leeks, carrots and seitan in the oil for

8–10 minutes, stirring occasionally. Add the cauliflower, miso and 200ml/7fl oz (UK)/scant 1C (US) of the water and simmer for a further 15 minutes or until the cauliflower is soft but firm. Squeeze out the juice from the grated ginger using your hands and add to the saucepan together with the tamari. Place the kuzu in a bowl, combine with 2 tbsps water and stir until dissolved. Add to the saucepan, mix for a few minutes until the sauce has thickened, then take off the heat. Serve with the rice.

### Tempeh, Almond and Broccoli Stir-Fry
*Serves 4–6*

*A simple stir-fry that goes well served with wholegrain noodles.*

INGREDIENTS
300g/11oz broccoli, broken into florets
5tbsp untoasted sesame oil
1 onion, peeled and chopped
225g/8oz tempeh, cubed
150g/5oz red cabbage, finely sliced
25g/1oz almonds, blanched
2tsp (UK)/2tsp (US) toasted sesame oil
3tbsp (UK)/¼C (US) tamari or soya sauce

Steam the broccoli florets for 8 minutes and set aside. Pour the untoasted sesame oil into a saucepan, add the onion and tempeh and sauté for 5 minutes or until the tempeh has begun to brown. Stir frequently to prevent burning. Add the red cabbage, almonds and toasted sesame oil and continue to fry until the cabbage softens. Stir in the tamari or soya sauce and broccoli, keep on the heat for another few minutes, then serve immediately.

**Tofu Mushroom Hats**
*Serves 4*

INGREDIENTS
4 large flat mushrooms
1 shallot, trimmed
Half a red pepper, trimmed
50g/2oz celery
1 clove of garlic, peeled and crushed
4tbsp (UK)/⅓C (US) olive oil
300g/11oz plain, firm tofu mashed
1tsp (UK)/1tsp (US) paprika
¼tsp (UK)/¼tsp (US) vegetable bouillon[3]
1tsp (UK)/1tsp (US) miso
4 heaped tbsp chopped fresh flat-leaf parsley

Peel the mushrooms, removing and reserving the stalks, and steam them for a couple of minutes. Place on an oiled baking tray.

For the filling, finely chop the mushroom stalks, shallot, red pepper and celery and sauté with the garlic in the olive oil for 5 minutes. Add the tofu, paprika, vegetable bouillon, miso and parsley and continue to heat for about another 5 minutes until all the ingredients are soft and well blended. Fill each mushroom with the tofu mixture and bake at 190°C/375°F/Gas 5 for 15 minutes.

**Cheese, Bean and Spinach Pancakes**
*Serves 6*

PANCAKE INGREDIENTS
100g/4oz wholemeal or spelt flour
sea salt and black pepper
1 free-range egg, beaten
225ml/8fl oz (UK)/1C (US) soya milk
1tsp (UK)/1tsp (US) olive oil

FILLING INGREDIENTS
200g/7oz cannellini beans, soaked overnight
1 strip of kombu, rehydrated
2tbsp (UK)/3tbsp (US) olive oil
300g/11oz leeks, trimmed and chopped
2 heaped tbsp black mustard seeds
½tsp (UK)/½tsp (US) vegetable bouillon
450g/1lb spinach, trimmed and chopped
100g/4oz vegetarian goat's Cheddar or firm soya cheese, grated
sea salt and black pepper

FILLING
Drain the beans, rinse and simmer in boiling water with the kombu for about 1 hour or until soft. Discard the excess water and set aside.

  Place the olive oil in a large saucepan and sauté the leeks and mustard seeds, stirring frequently until the leeks are soft. Add the vegetable bouillon, beans and spinach, cover and leave to steam for a couple of minutes until the spinach has shrunk. Take off the heat and mash. Mix in the grated cheese, sea salt and black pepper and combine all the ingredients well. Leave to one side.

PANCAKES
To make the pancakes, place the flour, sea salt and black pepper in a bowl, add the egg and soya milk and whisk. If the mixture develops lumps, put it briefly through a blender until smooth. Place 1 tsp of olive oil in a frying pan and gently heat. Add about 3tbsp (UK)/¼C (US) of the pancake batter to the pan, swirl it about so that mixture is even, and cook on either side for a couple of minutes until light, golden brown. Repeat until the batter is all used up (should make about 6 pancakes).

Divide the filling between the pancakes and roll them up. Extra grated cheese can be sprinkled on top of each pancake before serving if desired.

**Baby Vegetables in a Leek and Pecan Nut Sauce**
*Serves 6*

INGREDIENTS
450g/1lb new potatoes
200g/7oz baby carrots
200g/7oz baby turnips
150g/5oz baby sweetcorn
150g/5oz leeks, trimmed and chopped
1tbsp (UK)/1½tbsp (US) olive oil
50g/2oz pecan nuts
1tsp (UK)/1tsp (US) mustard powder
1tsp (UK)/1tsp (US) coarse-grain mustard
200ml/7fl oz (UK)/scant 1C (US) soya milk
1 heaped tsp dried thyme
½tsp (UK)/½tsp (US) vegetable bouillon

Steam the potatoes and baby vegetables for 15 minutes until tender. Sauté the leeks in the olive oil for a few minutes, then place in a blender with all the other ingredients and whizz until smooth. Gently heat through and serve with the vegetables.

## Spring Vegetable Soup
*Serves 6*

INGREDIENTS
2 spring onions, trimmed and chopped
1tbsp (UK)/1½tbsp (US) olive oil
150g/5oz baby carrots, peeled and chopped
50g/2oz celery, trimmed and chopped
200g/7oz potatoes, peeled and chopped
900ml/1⅔pints (UK)/4C(US) water
5 fresh bay leaves
1 sprig of fresh thyme
5 fresh basil leaves
3 heaped tbsp chopped fresh flat-leaf parsley
100g/4oz red lentils
1tbsp (UK)/1½tbsp (US) vegetable bouillon
sea salt and black pepper

In a large saucepan, briefly sauté the spring onions in the olive oil, then add the carrots, celery and potato and continue to cook for a few minutes, stirring all the time. Add the water, herbs, lentils, vegetable bouillon, sea salt and black pepper, bring to the boil and simmer for 25 minutes until the ingredients are very soft.

## Carrot and Raisin Muffins
*Makes approx. 12 muffins*

INGREDIENTS
400g/14oz plain wholemeal flour or spelt flour, sieved
2 heaped tsp salt-free baking powder
200g/7oz raisins
300g/11oz carrots, peeled and grated
200ml/7fl oz (UK)/scant 1C (US) sunflower oil plus a little for oiling
4 free-range eggs, beaten
200ml/7fl oz (UK)/scant 1C (US) maple syrup
200ml/7fl oz (UK)/scant 1C (US) rice milk
2tsp natural lemon essence
1tsp (UK)/2tsp (US) natural vanilla extract
sea salt

Combine the flour, baking powder, raisins, carrots and oil in a basin. Mix the eggs with the other wet ingredients and salt and stir into the flour mixture. Mix well until a thick batter is formed. Oil a muffin tray and fill it. Place in a preheated oven and bake at 180°C/350°F/Gas 4 for 20 minutes or until lightly golden.

## Marzipan Carob Balls
*Serves 4–6*

INGREDIENTS
175/6oz ground almonds
75ml/3fl oz (UK)/⅓C (US) brown rice syrup
2tsp (UK)/2tsp (US) natural green food colouring
1tbsp (UK)/1tbsp (US) natural almond essence
One 100g/4oz bar of sugar-free carob

Blend the ground almonds, brown rice syrup, green food colouring and almond essence together until ingredients are well combined. Form into small balls (should make about 14) and set aside.

Break the carob bar into pieces and place them in a heat-resistant casserole lid, suspended over a saucepan of simmering water. Allow the carob to melt. Roll the marzipan balls in the melted carob and place them on a tray lined with greaseproof paper. Leave to cool then chill.

## Fruit and Nut Chews
*Serves 4–6*

INGREDIENTS
175g/6oz dried dates
250ml/8fl oz (UK)/1C (US) water
50g/2oz pecan nuts, chopped
2 heaped tsp tahini
2 heaped tbsp peanut butter

Cook the dates in the water for about 10 minutes until they are soft and all the liquid has been absorbed. Add the pecans, tahini and peanut butter and mix well. Leave to sit for about 30 minutes so that the mixture firms up, then form into balls or logs and chill.

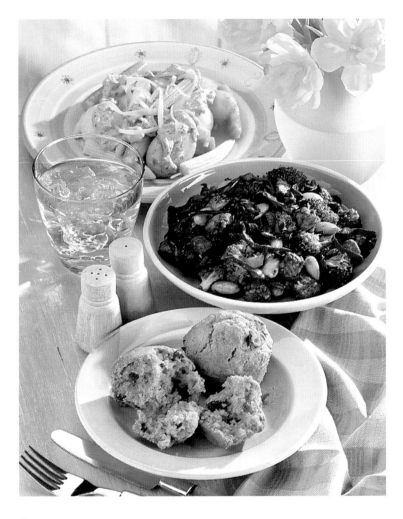

Spring:

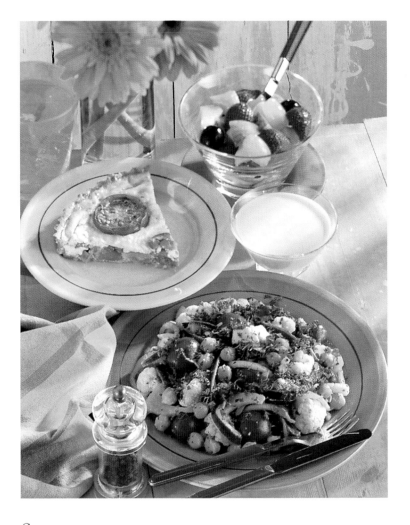

## Summer:

Cauliflower, Cherry Tomato and Red Onion Salad, *see* page 108
Asparagus, Tomato and Goat's Cheese Quiche, *see* page 111
Fresh Fruit Salad with Strawberry Crème, *see* page 117

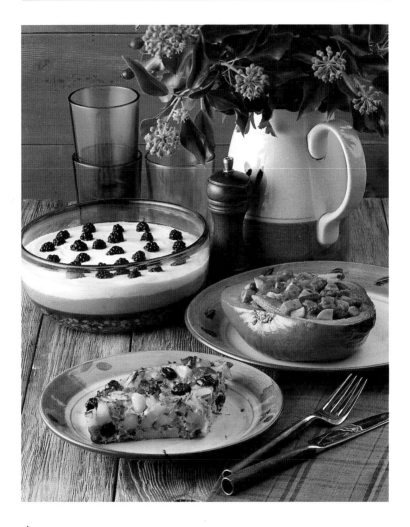

## Autumn:

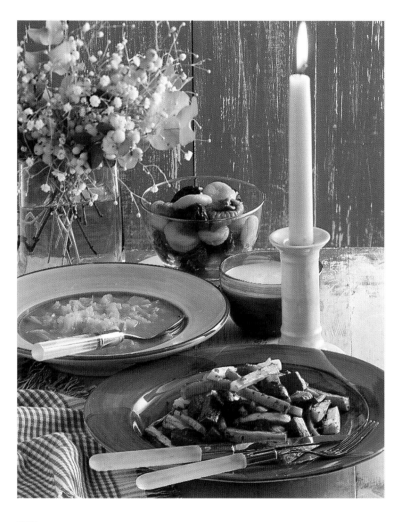

## Winter:

Spicy Winter Vegetable Soup, *see* page 174
Roast Root Salad, *see* page 165
Dried Fruit Compôt with Almond Whip, *see* page 176

# CHAPTER 7

# Summer

*O Summer sun, O moving trees!*
*O cheerful human noise, O busy glittering street!*
*What hour shall Fate in all the future find,*
*Or what delights, ever to equal these:*
*Only to taste the warmth, the light, the wind,*
*Only to be alive, and feel that life is sweet.*

LAURENCE BINYON

Spring merges into summer on 21 June, when we experience the longest amount of daylight of the year. This is known as the summer solstice.

During the summer, nature begins to bloom and manifest her magnificent glory. Colours of every hue surround us, activity climbs and the power of the sun is at its peak.

Many of us who live in a temperate zone look forward to this time of year. It's a season when we tend to spend more time out of doors, relaxing and soaking up the sunshine; rambling, cycling, playing tennis and caring for the garden are all amiable pastimes.

By exposing our bodies to the summer light, we can boost our immune systems; but of course it's wise to wear a protective sunscreen when outside at all times, and keep out of the sun's hottest rays, between 11 a.m. and 3 p.m.

The summer months are usually a good time to take holidays, allowing ourselves a break from life's continual demands. If we are travelling abroad, it's best to visit countries that are experiencing a similar climate or season to our own, so as not to confuse the body clock. However, if we're off to the other side of the world, this is unavoidable.

## A SUMMER DIET

In the summer we have the widest possible choice of food to pick from, as nature delivers her flourishing store. Leaves, stems, assorted green beans, herbs and fresh fruit are just some of the delicious plants available, making it a perfect season to take a bite into the raw.

The summer diet should be the lightest of all seasons. We can obtain our energy from cooling vegetables and succulent fruits, which will keep us well watered throughout the warm, dry days. Sprouts, tofu and tempeh are good sources of protein, being more suitable than the protein from animal produce. Whereas heavy flesh foods are heat-producing, sprouts and soya bean products, like most fruit and vegetables, have a cooling effect. In fact, for those who are not already vegetarian, the summer is a good time to make a transition.

Try to include foods that represent every earthly waking colour. Eat the reds of cherries and tomatoes, the oranges of carrots and nectarines, the greens of cucumbers, courgettes and peas, the yellows of peppers and peaches and the mauves and blues of aubergine and grapes. Each colour found in nature not only nourishes the body with its rainbow of pigments, but also helps cleanse and balance the more subtle energies of the chakra system (invisible, revolving vortexes of energy that are situated from the base of the spine to the top of the head and function as a pathway for the life force).

Summertime breakfasts needn't be too rich. Often a few pieces of fruit or some seeds and nuts and a large glass of mixed vegetable juice is sufficient. However people involved in physically laborious jobs or those with hypoglycaemic tendencies are likely to need something with a few more calories.

Other meals can consist of thickly filled wholemeal baps, grain risottos, stir-fries, stuffed vegetables and chilled soups, and with so many seasonal vegetables around it's possible to come up with a unique tasting salad each new day. Stuffed vegetables are one of my great favourites; besides rice, use other grains mixed with sautéed onions, tofu or nuts and fresh herbs to stuff tomatoes, peppers, aubergines, artichokes and courgettes.

*Suitable sandwiches*

With summer conjuring up antics of long days out, it's always practical to pack something healthy and satisfying to tag along. Sandwiches are consistently faithful furnishings and can be easily bundled into a bag or rucksack, just in case of an appetite attack. The humble sandwich can be a great source of energy, and with a little culinary inspiration will never become a bore.

So forget the cheese and pickle and egg mayonnaise, here are ten mouth-watering samples to take on tour or trek.

1 Lettuce, smoked or marinated tofu, mangetout, red onion rings and tofu mayonnaise.
2 Tabbouleh (see recipe below), hummus and vegetarian sausage.
3 Alfalfa, avocado and tomato.
4 Avocado, red pepper and coleslaw (see page 108 for a healthy coleslaw recipe).
5 Feta cheese, grated carrot, sun-dried tomato and tofu mayonnaise.
6 Goat's or tofu cheese, peach slices and grapes.
7 Scrambled egg or tofu, mushrooms and tamari.
8 Banana, date and tahini.
9 Mashed refried beans, tofu cheese, lettuce, cucumber and tomato.
10 Vegetable pâté, felafel and salad.

## Tabbouleh

250g/9oz bulgar wheat
200ml/7fl oz (UK)/scant 1C (US) tomato or mixed vegetable juice
3 ripe tomatoes, finely chopped
2 spring onions, finely chopped
50g/2oz finely chopped flat-leaf parsley
4 heaped tbsp finely chopped fresh mint
2tbsp (UK)/3tbsp (US) olive oil
2tbsp (UK)/3tbsp (US) lemon juice

Simmer the bulgar wheat in just under twice the volume of water until almost soft, then add the tomato or mixed vegetable juice and continue to heat until all the liquid has been absorbed. Remove from the heat, add the remaining ingredients and mix.

*Luscious leaves*

From the frilly lollo biondo to the peppery rocket, summer leaves make the perfect base to a host of seasonal salads. Being more than 90 per cent water they contain practically no calories, but fair amounts of the antioxidant vitamins A, C and E, plus folic acid, calcium and iron. Lettuce is also a sound remedy for insomnia, due to a compound known as lactucarium, which calms the nervous system and induces sleep. To help promote a good night's rest, drink a glass of lettuce juice half an hour before retiring.

Besides the common cos and the everyday Iceberg, try crinkly frisée, purple radicchio and mild endive – or any other local leaves that can be spotted. Layer them into sandwiches, use them as a bed for beans and grains or serve them on their own as an accompaniment to a main meal.

As summer is the season for salads, here are five summery dressings to trickle over those luscious leaves. Most dressings have a high oil content, so use them sparingly.

## Minty Yoghurt Dressing

*This is good with cucumber or tomatoes*

300ml/½ pint (UK)/1¼C (US) goat's yoghurt
2 heaped tsp chopped fresh basil
1 heaped tbsp chopped fresh mint
a pinch of dried dill
a pinch of black pepper

## Tomato and Chive Glaze

4tbsp (UK)/⅓C (US) tomato juice
4tbsp (UK)/⅓C (US) olive oil
1tsp (UK)/1tsp (US) lemon juice
1 heaped tbsp finely chopped chives
1tsp (UK)/1tsp (US) paprika

## Tarragon Walnut Dressing

4tbsp (UK)/⅓C (US) safflower oil
2tbsp (UK)/3tbsp (US) walnut oil
2tbsp (UK)/3tbsp (US) cider vinegar
2 heaped tbsp finely chopped fresh tarragon or 2 heaped tsp dried
tarragon

## Spicy Avocado Dressing

1 large ripe avocado
2 ripe tomatoes
1tbsp (UK)/1½tbsp (US) lemon juice
1tbsp (UK)/1½tbsp (US) olive oil
½ heaped tsp mild chilli powder
1 heaped tsp finely chopped onion

Place all the ingredients in a blender and whizz.

**Sunflower and Mustard Dressing**

4tbsp (UK)/⅓C (US) sunflower oil
4 heaped tbsp chopped fresh parsley
1tsp (UK)/1tsp (US) wholegrain mustard
1tsp (UK)/1tsp (US) brown rice vinegar
sea salt and black pepper

# JUICE

Having already tapped into the wonderful world of juices in Chapter 6, the sunny months from June to September allow us to become a little more acquainted. So here's an easy-to-access table of common vegetable saps.

*Figure 11, The nutrients and healing properties of ten vegetable juices*

| Vegetable juice | Nutrients | Healing properties |
| --- | --- | --- |
| Beetroot | Vitamin C, sodium, potassium, calcium, magnesium, manganese, chromium, nickel, chlorine. | General tonic, aids peristaltic action of intestines. Flushes out liver and gall bladder. Is a good blood-builder when mixed with other juices. |
| Cabbage | Beta-carotene, vitamin C, calcium, potassium, sulphur, iron, selenium. | Due to the presence of a substance known as vitamin U, cabbage juice hastens the healing of stomach and duodenal ulcers. It also appeases varicose veins, destroys internal parasites and can be applied externally to leg ulcers and wounds. |
| Carrot | Beta-carotene, vitamins B and C, sodium, potassium, calcium, magnesium, iron, chromium, iodine, cobalt, nickel. | Aids the respiratory and digestive systems, helps ward off colds and brightens the eyes. A good remedy for poor night vision. |

| Vegetable juice | Nutrients | Healing properties |
|---|---|---|
| Celery | Vitamin B and C, sodium, potassium, calcium, magnesium. | Removes excess fluid from the body (due to high organic sodium content which displaces inorganic sodium from the cells), is a strong alkalizer (neutralizing acid conditions), helps lower high blood pressure and is anti-inflammatory. |
| Cucumber | Potassium, sulphur, chlorine, silicon, manganese. | A mild diuretic, quenches the thirst, cools inflammatory conditions such as a sore throat, burning skin and irritated eyes. Rich silicon content improves skin quality. Possesses a protein-digesting enzyme called erepsis. |
| Lettuce | Beta-carotene, folic acid, PABA, silicon, sulphur. | Contains the sedative lactucarium which calms the nerves and impedes insomnia. It's also a mild diuretic and cools the body in hot weather. |
| Onion | Vitamins B and C, sodium, potassium, calcium, magnesium, iron, zinc, manganese, chromium, selenium, iodine, nickel. | Helps dispel worms from intestines, rids the body of colds, coughs and catarrh, contains a natural cholesterol fighter and inhibits the growth of cancerous cells. |
| Potato | Vitamin C, B complex, calcium, potassium, iron. | Reduces fluid retention and soothes the digestive tract. Possesses a natural antibiotic which helps promote bowel flora. Also contains abscisic acid, a natural plant hormone that enhances immunity. |
| Radish | Vitamin C, sodium, potassium, magnesium, calcium. | Strengthens mucous membranes, clears mucus from sinuses, cleans the liver, breaks up gall, kidney and bladder stones, soothes a sore throat, takes down abdominal swelling and purifies the blood. |
| Watercress | Beta-carotene, vitamin C, potassium, calcium, magnesium, sulphur, iron. | Good for the gall bladder and liver, is a blood builder and blood purifier as well. |

Some of the juices, such as onion, radish and watercress, become very condensed once juiced, so are best mixed with other, less potent juices or diluted with water. Carrot is an excellent base for any of these vegetables. For children, juices must always be diluted with equal amounts of water.

**Juicing equipment**

Before we travel on, I'd like to comment on juicing equipment. At present there are three main types of household juicers on the market: centrifugal, masticating and hydraulic.

*Centrifugal*

Centrifugal juicers run on electricity at high speed and are at the bottom of the price range. Fruit and vegetables are simply pushed through a revolving blade, where they are grated, separating juice from pulp. A centrifugal juicer is a good buy for the beginner.

*Masticating*

Masticating juicers such as the 'Champion' operates by mashing the fruit and vegetables before pressing them through a stainless-steel sieve. Although these juicers are more expensive than the centrifugal styles (approximately £350/$550), they extract a much greater percentage of juice and in the long run are cost-efficient.

*Hydraulic*

The hydraulic juice press works by cutting up fresh produce to a fine pulp and then pressing it under high pressure through a woven nylon cloth. The hydraulic technique is a cut above the masticating models, removing all juice and rendering a moisture-less pulp. Those juicing for therapeutic reasons are advised to go for the masticating or hydraulic juicer, as the more juice that is squeezed from a plant the richer in nutrients the juice will be.

With centrifugal juicers, instead of throwing away the pulp left over you can add it to savouries, bakes and veg burgers.

Most juicers run on electricity, and the electrical current can cause an energy exchange to occur within the cells of the expelled material. To correct this polarity jump a small piece of clear quartz crystal can be briefly placed into the juice just after extraction.

## HEALING HERBS

*'A good kitchen is a good Apothecaries shop'*
WILLIAM BULLEIN

Another delicious treat that awaits us in the summer is the generous diversity of fresh and fragrant herbs. They're a fabulous substitute for the salt shaker, their delicate aromas adding gusto to many a meal. When using herbs in cooking, it's best to introduce them to the dish just before the food is ready. This prevents the needless destruction of their nutrients and preserves their flavour and colour too. To make original home-made herb vinegars, infuse fresh herbs in cider vinegar for a couple of weeks.

Besides tantalizing our taste buds, culinary herbs are renowned for their numerous healing properties. As the amount added to food preparation is limited, for therapeutic results they can be brewed up into teas and drunk three times a day.

### How to make a medicinal tea

Place 50g/2oz of fresh herbs or 25g/1oz of dried into a saucepan, pour over 600ml/1 pint of boiling water and cover. Let steep for 10–15 minutes. Then strain and drink. For coarser parts of the herb such as stems, roots and barks, simmering the ingredients for 10–20 minutes will allow the goodness to be released. Herbal infusions can last up to three days when stored in a fridge.

*Figure 12, Ten culinary herbs that heal*

| Herb | Healing properties | Culinary uses |
| --- | --- | --- |
| Basil | Helps combat colds, fevers and the flu, strengthens the kidneys and bladder. Has an all-over tonic effect. | Add to salads, tomato dishes, pasta, soups and sauces. |
| Coriander leaf (also known as cilantro or Chinese lettuce) | Relieves urinary tract infections, rids gas from the bowel. | Add to salads, soups, curries, stir-fries. |
| Dill (also known as dill weed) | Contains carvone, a compound that reduces intestinal gas. | Add to breads, dips and salad dressings. |
| Marjoram | Eases headaches, stomach cramps and nervous complaints. A good pick-me-up. | Add to casseroles, stews, bakes, potatoes, summer squash. |
| Mint | Alleviates indigestion, nausea and flatulence. | Add to green salads, summer vegetables , potatoes and desserts. |
| Oregano | Enhances digestion and helps clear coughs and colds. | Add to salads, casseroles, pizza, pasta sauces, soups and other savouries. |
| Parsley | Breath freshener, mild diuretic, fortifies digestive and respiratory systems. Also treats urinary tract infections. | Add to soups, salads, entrées – almost everything. |
| Rosemary | Use as an aspirin alternative. Calms the nervous system, boosts digestion. Externally, the cool infusion can be massaged into the scalp to improve hair and scalp condition. | Add to baked vegetables, soups and hot-pots. |
| Sage | Reduces excessive pespiration, night sweats and hot flushes. Halts the flow of breast milk. Soothes the throat and abates respiratory conditions. Like rosemary, the cool infusion can be applied as a hair and scalp tonic. | Add to soups, sauces, casseroles, veg burgers and bakes. |
| Thyme | Lessens symptoms of bronchitis, whooping cough and other respiratory maladies. Can also be used as a gargle for the mouth. | Add to salads, soups, stews, sauces and bakes. |

# FRUIT

*The fruit of the trees shall be for meat and the leaf thereof for medicine.*

from EZEKIEL 47:12

Summer is the most obvious season in which to tuck into a spectrum of juicy, ripe fruits. Not only do they hydrate and cleanse, but they also keep us feeling cool and refreshed throughout the summer. Fruit is at its best when it has been left to ripen naturally on the vine or tree, in the sun. This is so the starch inside the fruit can be converted into an easily digestible fruit sugar. Local, seasonal fruits are not usually picked until ripe, whereas imported produce is often plucked prematurely. This is so it doesn't spoil by the time it reaches its destination – another reason for opting for food that's home grown! If unripe fruit is purchased, it should be left to ripen at room temperature. To do this, place it in a brown paper bag and store in a dark place for two to three days. Apples, grapes, berries and citrus fruit do not ripen once picked and should be considered inedible if not fully matured.[1] Exotic fruits should only be eaten in season by people living in tropical climates.

Those who are allergic to aspirin (made from a synthetic substance called salicylic acid), may need to watch their intake of salicylate-rich fruits. These include blackberries, blueberries, cherries, currants, dates, oranges, prunes, raspberries and straw-berries; all exhibit salicylate-like activity.

However, this batch of foods may be a blessing in disguise. Eaten on a regular basis, they are believed to demonstrate similar protective qualities to that of aspirin, benefiting headache sufferers and casualties of heart disease without the potential side-effects.

To put fruits in their rightful places, they can be divided into five main groups (exotic fruits are marked with an asterisk):

*Acid fruits*

These are cranberries, gooseberries, grapefruit, lemons, limes, loganberries, oranges, pineapple*, sour plums, satsumas, strawberries, tangerines, tomatoes.

The acid-fruit category does not mean that these fruits are acid-forming. The acid present leaves the body soon after ingestion (with the exception of cranberries and sour plums), resulting in an alkaline ash. Sometimes these acids can aggravate an already over-acidic state, eg in those with rheumatism or arthritis. In such cases, acid fruits, especially citrus, should be limited.

*Sub-acid fruits*

These are apples, apricots, blackberries, blackcurrants, blueberries, boysenberries, cherries, elderberries, figs (fresh), grapes, kiwi*, nectarines, peaches, pears, plums, raspberries.

All sub-acid fruits are alkaline-forming.

*Sweet fruits*[2]

These are bananas*, dates, sweet grapes, mangoes*, papayas*, dried fruit.

Fruits in the sweet fruit group contain the richest amount of natural sugars, making them the most energy-giving of all fruits.

*Melons*

These are the cantaloupe, honeydew, watermelon, etc.

Melons are digested exceedingly quickly in the small intestine and should therefore be eaten strictly on their own.

*Avocados and olives*

Although we may not perceive avocados and olives as fruits, botanically they fit into this classification. But whilst most fruit is low in fat and calories, these two are quite the opposite. Both are fairly concentrated in monounsaturated oils and are a notable source of the fat-soluble vitamins A and E.

## Feasting on fruit

Fruit makes a handsome snack in between meals or quite a meal in itself. Chop up some apricots, peaches and nectarines, add some strawberries, cherries and grapes, and take pleasure in a bowl full of heavenly pickings. Although most fruits are best eaten on their own (to prevent internal fermentation), as a treat they can be whizzed up in yoghurt or soya cream, or blended with oat milk and nuts into sensational smoothies. To become better versed in our favourite fruits, here are eight fruitful secrets unveiled.

- Apples contain a soluble fibre called pectin that tones intestinal muscles and helps reduce high blood cholesterol. Pectin also latches on to heavy metals in the body and carries them out of the system. Although other fruits contain pectin apple fibre has the most stabilizing effect on blood-sugar levels, and, because of their properties, apples are used in many studies researching cholesterol reduction. Malic acid, another constituent of apples, destroys disease-producing bacteria in the digestive tract.
- Berries are rich in capillary-strengthening flavonoids. Active substances found in bilberries have been linked to the prevention of cataracts and glaucoma and also to the improvement of night vision. The astringent properties of blueberries (dried) rectify diarrhoea and strawberries contain ellagic acid, an anti-cancer compound that neutralizes the damaging effects of cigarette smoke.
- Cherries, like most berries, are rich in capillary-enhancing flavonoids and are a good source of iron. They also help cleanse the liver and gall bladder and relieve the symptoms of rheumatism and gout.
- Cranberries (berries that deserve a mention of their own),

although one of the rare acid-forming fruits, are a marvellous medicine for bladder infections (cystitis). They contain a component that interferes with the adherence of bacteria to the lining of the urinary tract and also possess anti-bacterial properties.

For medicinal purposes, cranberries can be juiced and taken several times a day. Combining them with sweeter fruits such as grapes will smooth over their bitter taste.

- Grapefruit eaten before a meal stimulates the appetite by arousing the digestive juices. It also contains a soluble fibre called galacturonic acid that reduces arterial plaque.
- Grapes are a great natural laxative, their high potassium and magnesium content being the reason for their top cleansing abilities. In fact, fasting on grapes has become a well-known self-helper in treating cancer and other serious illnesses. Red grapes contain more iron than green.
- Lemons contain both antiseptic and anti-microbial properties and are therefore effective in the treatment of mild infections. A sore throat or bout of flu responds well to the intake of this fruit. The lemon also seems to be able to increase elimination through the skin, helping to reduce the symptoms of a high temperature. Dilute the juice of one lemon in a cup of hot water, add a little honey and sip.
- Pears, similar to apples, contain potent pectin, the cholesterol bludger. They also stimulate digestion and possess anti-inflammatory actions.

**Food combining**

Having looked at fruit, foods that in most circumstances are better digested alone, we shall now put the theory and application of friendly foods together and focus on the art of 'food combining'.

Food combining, often referred to as the 'Hay' diet (the Hay system was first introduced by Dr William Howard Hay, 1866–1940), is the practice of mixing – or not mixing – specific foods at the same meal. This is so that optimum digestion can be achieved. To accomplish this, it's recommended that carbo-hydrate (starch), which requires an alkaline medium for its breakdown, should not be consumed with protein, which requires an acid medium.

Although the routine of separating conflicting food groups has helped a host of people overcome a heap of health problems, I prefer to cover this practice with a non-extremist view.

Basically, those who follow a vegetarian diet and steer clear of processed junk on the whole do not need to worry too much about the rules. Plant-based foods, especially when eaten raw, contain their own specific digestive enzymes that aid assimilation, whatever the internal environment. This means that vegetarian protein sources such as seeds and nuts should be able to be happily blended with starchy grains and beans.

Those who continue to consume the unnecessary high protein contained in animal produce can definitely benefit by eating their protein away from starch. Flesh foods take far longer to digest than carbohydrates and entail a lot of hard work. When meat or eggs are eaten with starchy foods, the outcome is a clash in digestive juices and an insufficient production of the appropriate enzymes. This results in indigestion, bloating and fatigue.

To turn the rather complicated system of food combining into a more accessible guide, here are some suggestions to put into action.

- Omnivores are advised not to mix protein and starch at the same meal. This means not eating meat, poultry, fish or eggs with grains, legumes, potatoes or winter squash.
- Those following a plant-based diet who experience symptoms of heartburn, bloating or gas, or are prone to food-induced allergic reactions, may benefit from consuming their protein and carbohydrate at separate meals. Vegetable sources of protein include nuts and seeds; grains, potatoes, legumes and winter squash are classed as starch.
- Vegetables (besides potatoes and winter squash) are compatible when eaten with protein or carbohydrates.
- Most fruit, due to its quicker-than-quick breakdown, is best

eaten as a separate food group. The exceptions are acid fruits, which can be combined freely with seeds, nuts and goat's milk produce, and avocados and olives, which are neutral and go well with everything.

- Do not drink whilst eating as this may cause a dilution in digestive enzymes. If possible allow one hour to elapse without fluids before and after meals.

### Summer cooking techniques

The most complementary way of enjoying food in this season is to place the emphasis on the raw. Uncooked vegetables, sprouts, fruit, seeds and nuts can make up a good 50–70 per cent of the diet (depending on individual needs) whilst the remainder can consist of boiled grains and other quick-cooked edibles.

One of the main plusses of eating our food in its raw state is that it's packed with live enzymes, the catalysts of life. Once these enzymes are liberated via the chewing process they immediately get to work, helping to break down the food that they were released from. This means that our digestive system doesn't have to work as hard – hence the importance of chewing our food well.

Sprouted seeds possess the greatest enzyme activity, followed by fresh fruit and vegetables and naturally fermented foods such as miso and tempeh.

Raw fruit and vegetables (whether organic or not, often harbour parasites and micro-organisms, invisible to the naked eye. Washing produce in water alone does not remove all of these unwanted particles. So here's a clean-up method that should do the job.

Soak all raw produce in a diluted solution of cider vinegar and water for 10 minutes. Rinse well. There are also several environmentally friendly fruit and vegetable washes on the market.

### Plant power

Other compounds found in raw foods that are often destroyed in the cooking process are known as phytochemicals. Unlike vitamins and minerals, these plant chemicals are not essential for life, but certainly offer many rewarding benefits.

We've already looked at one of them, chlorophyll the green blood-builder, in Chapter 6. So let's now uncover some of the other fascinating raw food factors.

*Flavonoids*

Flavonoids, of which there are several thousand, are a group of plant pigments that possess some remarkable healing possibilities.

First of all they have a tremendous augmenting power on blood capillaries, preventing and reversing circulatory afflictions. High blood pressure, bleeding gums, chilblains, haemorrhoids and varicose veins are some of the conditions where these compounds are indicated. Flavonoids also synergistically enhance the cellular absorption of vitamin C. In nature, where everything (if left untampered-with) exists in harmony, both substances are found hand in hand.

Two flavonoids that have been well documented in recent years are those found in many colourful summer fruits. These are known as anthocyanidins and proanthocyanidins and are sturdy scavengers of free radicals (unstable molecules produced within the body that may damage surrounding cells if left unchecked).

Such phytochemicals help promote synthesis of collagen, an elastic-like material responsible for the scaffolding of all body tissues. Furthermore, they work by restoring the flexibility of connective tissue, and greatly strengthen ligaments, tendons, cartilage, bones, teeth and blood vessels. As for anti-inflammatory and anti-allergic effects, the powerful pair restrain histamine and inflammatory prostaglandin release, substances associated with aversive responses.

Good food sources of flavonoids include buckwheat (for rutin), citrus fruit (hesperidin), berries, cherries and grapes (anthocyanidins and proanthocyanidins).

*Carotenoids*

The substances that lend fruit and vegetables their orange colour are known as carotenoids. It's now reported that there's a direct correlation between the increased amount of carotenoids stored in our body cells and the decreased incidence of benign tumours.

Lycopene, a carotenoid found richly concentrated in tomatoes, is considered to be one of nature's most powerful antioxidants and appears to protect against cancers of the mouth, pharynx, oesophagus, stomach, colon and prostate. Other carotenoids are found in large amounts in carrots, apricots, sweet potatoes, squash and all dark leafy greens, where the orange colouring is disguised by green chloroplast cells.

*Ellagic acid*

Strawberries, raspberries, grapes, apples and walnuts all contain an active antioxidant known as ellagic acid, which prevents the action of many cancer-forming pollutants harming the body.

*Indoles*

Indoles are compounds found in the Cruciferae family of vegetables and function to protect the body from cancer-causing agents. Cruciferous vegetables include broccoli, Brussels sprouts, cabbage, cauliflower, cress, kale, kohlrabi, radish, swede and turnip.

*Hormone helpers*

Animals aren't the only ones that rely on hormones. Plants, too, possess hormone-like substances that act as chemical messengers. Some of these have been found to help regulate our own hormonal system.

Soya beans, almonds, cashews, peanuts, oats, corn, wheat and apples all have traces of oestrogenic activity, oestrogen being a female hormone that gradually declines during and after the menopause.

Now since an excess of oestrogen in the body can predispose us to certain types of cancer (breast or prostate), it would be logical to believe that oestrogens in food would increase this risk. On the contrary, they actually do the reverse. This is because plant oestrogens bind with the dangerous-type oestrogens made in the body and mimic the hormone, without causing any detrimental effects.

## SUMMER REVIEW

1 Eat light.
2 Entertain raw foods.
3 Dig into the fruit bowl.
4 Go vegetarian.
5 Keep well hydrated.
6 Participate in outdoor activities.
7 Enjoy a well-earned holiday.

To conclude our visit to summer, here's a shopping guide to the fresh produce in season. It also includes a variety of dried wholefoods, which although aren't distinctly summery are essential store-cupboard provisions.

*Figure 13, Fresh foods in summer*

| Nuts | Grains | Seeds | Sprouts |
|------|--------|-------|---------|
| almonds | amaranth | hemp | All sprouted |
| Brazil nuts | barley | linseeds | legumes, grains |
| cashews | buckwheat | pumpkin | and seeds |
| chestnuts | bulgar wheat | sesame | |
| hazelnuts | maize | sunflower | |
| macadamia | millet | | |
| peanuts | oats | | |
| pecans | rice | | |
| pine nuts | wheat | | |
| pistachios | wild rice | | |
| walnuts | quinoa | | |

*Figure 13, Fresh foods in summer* (cont.)

| Vegetables | Fruit | Herbs | Beans/Pulses |
|---|---|---|---|
| asparagus | apricots | basil | adzuki |
| aubergines or | avocados | bay | black turtle |
| eggplants | blackberries | chervil | black-eyed |
| beetroot | blackcurrants | chives | borlotti |
| broccoli | blueberries | coriander leaf | broad |
| cabbage | cherries | dill (also known | cannellini |
| carrots | damsons | as dill weed) | chickpeas |
| cauliflower | gooseberries | marjoram | field |
| celeriac | grapes | mint | flageolet |
| celery | loganberries | oregano | haricot |
| Chinese leaves | melons | parsley | mung |
| courgettes or | nectarines | rosemary | pinto |
| zucchini | peaches | sage | red kidney |
| cress | pears | savory | soya |
| cucumber | plums | tarragon | lentils |
| fennel | rhubarb | thyme | split peas |
| globe artichokes | strawberries | | |
| green beans | citrus fruit | | |
| horseradish | | | |
| lettuce | | | |
| mooli | | | |
| mushrooms | | | |
| onions | | | |
| peas | | | |
| peppers | | | |
| potatoes | | | |
| mangetout | | | |
| radishes | | | |
| spinach | | | |
| sweetcorn | | | |
| Swiss chard | | | |
| tomatoes | | | |
| watercress | | | |

# SUMMER RECIPES

## Mixed Sprout, Watercress and Avocado Salad
*Serves 4–8*

*This salad is delicious served without a dressing except for the lemon juice, which prevents the avocado from discolouring.*

INGREDIENTS
50g/2oz of mixed sprouts, eg mung beans, lentils, chickpeas
50g/2oz alfalfa sprouts
One 100g/4oz box of mustard and cress, trimmed
25g/1oz watercress, trimmed
75g/2½oz radish, trimmed and sliced
250g/9oz cucumber, peeled
1 large avocado, peeled
1 red pepper, deseeded
25g/1oz chives
1 tbsp (UK)/1½tbsp (US) lemon juice

Place the sprouted legumes, alfalfa, mustard and cress, watercress and radish in a salad bowl. Chop the cucumber, avocado, red pepper and chives into small pieces and add to the other ingredients. Stir in the lemon juice and gently combine. Refrigerate until required.

## Cauliflower, Cherry Tomato and Red Onion Salad
*Serves 6–8*

INGREDIENTS
100g/4oz chickpeas, soaked overnight
1 strip of kombu, rehydrated
1 small cauliflower, trimmed and cut into small florets
400g/14oz cherry tomatoes, halved
1 red onion, peeled and finely sliced
100g/4oz fennel, trimmed and finely sliced
6 heaped tbsp chopped parsley
Dressing
1tbsp (UK)/1½tbsp (US) sunflower oil
2tsp (UK)/2tsp (US) wholegrain mustard
1tbsp (UK)/1½tbsp (US) white miso
½tsp (UK)/½tsp (US) clear honey or brown rice syrup
sea salt and black pepper

Drain and rinse the chickpeas. Simmer in boiling water with the kombu for about 1½–2 hours or until soft. Remove excess water and set aside.

Add the cauliflower, tomatoes, red onion, fennel and parsley to the chickpeas and combine. Mix the dressing ingredients together, pour over the salad and stir.

## Crunchy Nut Coleslaw
*Serves 4–8*

INGREDIENTS
200g/7oz white cabbage, finely shredded
200g/7oz red cabbage, finely shredded
400g/14oz carrots, peeled and grated
3 spring onions, trimmed and chopped
100g/4oz pecan nuts, halved
50g/2oz seedless raisins
200ml/7fl oz (UK)/scant 1C (US) thick goat's or soya yoghurt
1tbsp (UK)/1½tbsp (US) cider vinegar
sea salt and black pepper

Combine the cabbages, carrots, spring onions, nuts and raisins in a bowl. Stir in the yoghurt and cider vinegar and add salt and pepper to taste.

**Green Bean, Arame and Coriander Salad**
*Serves 4–6*

INGREDIENTS
2 heaped tbsp arame seaweed
50g/2oz small white mushrooms, cleaned and sliced
1½tbsp (UK)/2tbsp (US) sesame oil
300g/11oz dwarf beans, trimmed and chopped
200g/7oz celery, trimmed and chopped
50g/2oz pitted black olives
150g/5½oz marinated tofu,[3] cubed
4 heaped tbsp finely chopped fresh coriander
¼ heaped tsp dried paprika
sea salt

Soak the arame in boiling water for 5 minutes, drain and set aside. Fry the mushroom in 1tbsp (UK)/1½tbsp (US) of the sesame oil for a few minutes and place in a salad bowl. Steam the dwarf beans for 10 minutes until soft and add to the mushrooms. Mix in the celery, olives, tofu, coriander, arame, the remaining oil, paprika and salt and gently combine.

**Savoury Courgette Boats**
*Makes 8 boats*

INGREDIENTS
4 courgettes or zucchini, trimmed and sliced in half lengthways
1 onion, peeled and chopped
2tbsp (UK)/3tbsp (US) olive oil
1 clove of garlic, peeled and crushed
1 heaped tsp black mustard seeds
3tbsp (UK)/¼C (US) tomato puree
200g/7oz bulgar wheat
500ml/16fl oz (UK)/2C (US) water
1tsp (UK)/1tsp (US) vegetable bouillon
1 heaped tbsp dried dill
1 heaped tsp yellow mustard powder
sea salt and freshly ground black pepper
50g/2oz vegetarian goat's Cheddar or firm soya cheese, grated

Steam the zucchini or courgettes for 8 minutes, then leave to cool. Once cool, remove the inner flesh, taking care not to damage the outer skin, and set both skin and flesh aside.

In a saucepan, sauté the onion in the olive oil until transparent. Add the garlic and mustard seeds and continue to fry for a few minutes, stirring frequently. Mix in the bulgar wheat and 2tbsp (UK)/3tbsp (US) of the tomato purée and continue to stir until all the oil has been absorbed. Then pour on the water, vegetable bouillon, dill, mustard powder, the reserved inner flesh from the zucchini or courgettes, salt and pepper and simmer for a further 15 minutes.

Once the bulgar is soft and all the water has been absorbed, add half of the grated cheese and mix together. Stuff the zucchini or courgette hollows with the grain mixture, sprinkling the remaining cheese on top. Bake in a preheated oven at 190°C/375°F/Gas 5 for 10 minutes. Serve immediately.

**Asparagus, Tomato and Goat's Cheese Quiche**
*Serves 6–8*

PASTRY INGREDIENTS
sunflower oil for oiling
100g/4oz plain wholemeal or spelt flour, sieved
sea salt
50g/2oz unhydrogenated sunflower margarine
3tbsp (UK)/¼C (US) water

FILLING INGREDIENTS
150g/5oz asparagus, trimmed and chopped
2 tomatoes, sliced
100g/4oz vegetarian goat's Cheddar, grated
2 free-range eggs, beaten
1 heaped tsp mustard powder
300ml/½ pint (UK)/1¼C (US) plain soya milk
sea salt and black pepper

Oil a 20cm/8in round flan dish and set aside. Place the flour, salt and margarine in a basin and rub together until the mixture resembles breadcrumbs. Add the water and mix into a dough. The pastry can be left to rest for 20 minutes. Using a rolling pin, roll out the pastry and place in the oiled dish. Bake in a preheated oven at 205°C/400°F/Gas 6 for 10 minutes.

Steam the asparagus for 10 minutes and arrange evenly on the pastry crust. Cover with a layer of half the sliced tomatoes, followed by the cheese. Combine the eggs, mustard powder, soya milk, salt and pepper and mix well. Pour into the pastry case, add a second layer of tomatoes decoratively just underneath the surface of the mixture and return to the oven. Bake for 30–35 minutes or until set and slightly golden. This dish is probably better eaten warm rather than hot and it can also be eaten cold.

**Baby Pimento Pizzas**
*Makes 8 pizzas*

PIZZA BASE
225g/8oz plain wholemeal flour, sieved
1 heaped tsp salt-free baking powder
¼ heaped tsp sea salt
1tbsp (UK)/1½tbsp (US) sunflower or olive oil and extra for oiling
150ml/¼ pint (UK) 1⅔C (US) water

TOMATO SAUCE
Half an onion, peeled and finely chopped
1tbsp (UK)/1½tbsp (US) sunflower oil
1 clove garlic, peeled and crushed
50g/2oz carrots, peeled and finely grated
150ml/¼ pint (UK)/⅔C (US) tomato or mixed vegetable juice
4tbsp (UK)/⅓C (US) tomato purée
1 heaped tsp dried oregano
2 heaped tsp dried basil
sea salt

CHEEZE SAUCE
One 400g/14oz can of red pimentos, drained
100g/4oz sunflower seeds
1 heaped tsp dried dill
1tsp (UK)/1tsp (US) lemon juice
1 heaped tbsp chopped onion
Half a clove of garlic
sea salt
100g/4oz cashew nuts

TOPPING
Half an onion, peeled and finely chopped
1 green pepper, deseeded and finely chopped
50g/2oz pitted black olives, chopped

Lightly oil a large baking tray and set aside. In a large bowl combine the flour, baking powder and salt and mix well. Add the oil and water, mixing until all the ingredients are moistened. Work into a dough with hands and knead for 5 minutes. Divide the mixture into eight pieces, rolling into small balls. Then, using a rolling pin, roll each ball out into a mini-pizza base measuring about 12cm/4½ in across.

Heat a dry, non-stick skillet on a low flame and cook each base on either side for about a minute or until slightly golden. Once cooked, place on the oiled baking tray.

To prepare the tomato sauce, sauté the onion in the oil until transparent. Add the garlic and carrot and continue to sauté until the vegetables are fairly soft. Then add the tomato or mixed vegetable juice and tomato purée and simmer for 10 minutes, stirring occasionally. Once cooked, mix in the herbs and salt.

For the cheeze sauce, place the pimentos in a liquidizer, add the sunflower seeds, dill, lemon juice, onion, garlic and salt and blend. Whilst blending, slowly add the cashew nuts, until a thick, smooth paste is formed.

Spread the tomato sauce in a thin layer over each pizza base. Then add a layer of the cheeze sauce. Finally mix vegetables for the topping together, sprinkle on and bake in a preheated oven at 180°C/350°F/ Gas 4 for 15 minutes.

## Wild Rice Paella Peppers
*Makes 8 peppers*

INGREDIENTS
4 large green peppers, deseeded and cut in half lengthways
150g/5oz long-grain brown rice
50g/2oz wild rice, soaked overnight
1 heaped tsp saffron
3tbsp (UK)/¼C (US) olive oil
1 onion, peeled and chopped
1 medium courgette or zucchini, trimmed and chopped
1 clove of garlic, peeled and crushed
50g/2oz tomatoes, chopped
50g/2oz broken cashew nuts
One 100g/4oz can of sweetcorn kernels, drained
100ml/4fl oz (UK)/½C (US) tomato juice
1 heaped tsp paprika
sea salt and black pepper
2tsp (UK)/2tsp (US) soya sauce

Steam the pepper halves for 5 minutes and place on a large baking tray. Cook the rice in twice the volume of water for 30 minutes, adding the saffron to the boiling water before the rice in order to rehydrate it first. The amount of water needed may vary according to brand of rice.

Place the olive oil in a saucepan and sauté the onion, zucchini or courgette and garlic until the onions are transparent. Add the tomatoes, cashews and sweetcorn and cook for a further few minutes. Then add the tomato juice, paprika, salt and pepper and leave to simmer for 10 minutes. Finally mix in the cooked rice and soya sauce and simmer until all the tomato juice has been absorbed. Fill each pepper half with rice mixture and bake in a preheated oven at 190°C/375°F/Gas 5 for 10 minutes.

## Basil, Spinach and Pine Nut Tagliatelle
*Serves 4–6*

INGREDIENTS
1 onion, peeled and chopped
1 clove of garlic, peeled and crushed
2tbsp (UK)/3tbsp (US) olive oil
100g/4oz tomatoes, chopped
1 bay leaf
1tsp (UK)/1tsp (US) vegetable bouillon
25g/1oz finely chopped fresh basil
25g/1oz pine kernels
1 heaped tsp dried basil
200g/7oz spinach, trimmed and chopped
200g/7oz wholemeal tagliatelle

In a saucepan, sauté the onion and garlic in the olive oil until the onion is transparent. Add the tomatoes, bay leaf and vegetable bouillon and simmer for 20 minutes. Stir in the fresh basil and continue to cook for a minute or so.

Remove the bay leaf and place the cooked vegetables with the pine kernels in a liquidizer and blend into a thick paste. Pour back into the saucepan, add the dried basil, mix and set aside.

Steam the spinach for 5 minutes, adding it to the basil sauce once cooked. Meanwhile cook the tagliatelle in boiling water until tender, drain well and serve immediately with the sauce.

## Roast Summer Vegetables in a Tofu and Horseradish Sauce
*Serves 6–8*

*A novel way to cook summer vegetables. The cauliflower and broccoli should remain slightly crisp.*

INGREDIENTS
1 medium aubergine or eggplant, trimmed and cut into wedges
450g/1lb broccoli, trimmed and broken into medium size florets
Sea salt
200ml/7fl oz (UK)/scant 1C (US) water
1tsp (UK)/1tsp (US) vegetable bouillon
1 fennel root, trimmed and sliced
1 medium cauliflower, trimmed and broken into florets
1 red pepper, deseeded and chopped into wedges
6tbsp (UK)/²/₃C (US) olive oil
Sauce
250g/9oz plain firm tofu, mashed
2 heaped tbsp finely grated wild horseradish
250ml/8fl oz (UK)/1C (US) water
1tsp (UK)/1tsp (US) white miso
3tbsp (UK)/¼C (US) sunflower oil
sea salt

Place the aubergine or eggplant in a bowl lined with kitchen paper, sprinkle over a little sea salt and leave to sit for 15 minutes. Then rinse.

Combine the water and the vegetable bouillon and pour into a large casserole or lasagne dish. Place the vegetables, including the aubergine or eggplant, inside the dish, brushing them all over with olive oil. Sprinkle on a little more salt, cover with foil and bake in a preheated oven at 205°C/400°F/Gas 6 for 50 minutes. Finally remove the foil and leave to roast for a further 5 minutes, taking care not to let the vegetables burn.

To prepare the sauce, blend half of the tofu with the horseradish, water, miso and oil together in a liquidizer. Add the remaining tofu and the salt and blend until smooth. Serve with the roasted vegetables.

**Fresh Fruit Salad with Strawberry Crème**
*Serves 6*

FRUIT SALAD
200g/7oz strawberries, halved
200g/7oz cherries
100g/4oz seedless white grapes
100g/4oz seedless red grapes
2 medium-size peaches, chopped
half a small melon, peeled and chopped

STRAWBERRY CRÈME
250g/9oz plain firm tofu
100ml/4fl oz (UK)/½C (US) apple juice
2tbsp (UK)/3tbsp (US) maize or brown rice syrup
1tbsp (UK)/1½tbsp (US) natural strawberry essence
½tsp (UK)/½tsp (US) natural vanilla essence
50ml/2fl oz sunflower oil

In a blender whizz together half of the tofu and all the other ingredients until smooth. Then add the remaining tofu and continue to blend. Place the crème in the fridge to chill. Meanwhile combine the fruit in a bowl and serve with the crème.

**Mint Carob Chip Tofu Ice Cream**
*Serves 6*

550g/1¼lb plain firm tofu
300ml/½pt (UK)/1¼C (US) rice milk
5tbsp (UK)/½C (US) maize or brown rice syrup
1tsp (UK)/1tsp (US) maple syrup
2tsp (UK)/2tsp (US) natural peppermint essence
1tbsp (UK)/1½tbsp (US) natural green food colouring
1tbsp (UK)/1½tbsp (US) natural vanilla essence
150ml/¼ pint (UK)/⅔C (US) sunflower oil
25g/1oz pecan nuts
One 150g/5oz carob bar, sugar-free

Blend all the ingredients except the carob bar until a thick cream is formed. Grate the carob bar and stir into the mixture, but do not blend. Pour into a plastic container and freeze. Defrost for half an hour before serving.


## Mocha Apricot and Hazelnut Whip
*Serves 6*

*A rich, creamy dessert that's a meal in itself. Also makes a great summer breakfast.*

300g/11oz dried apricots, soaked in water overnight
600ml/21fl oz (UK)/2¾C (US) apple juice
680g/1½lb plain firm tofu
2tbsp (UK)/3tbsp (US) maize or brown rice syrup
3 heaped tbsp hazelnut butter
100ml/4fl oz (UK)/½C (US) sunflower oil
6tbsp (UK)/⅔C (US) grain coffee substitute
1tsp (UK)/1tsp (US) natural vanilla essence
3tsp (UK)/4tsp (US) natural orange essence
3 heaped tbsp sugar-free apricot jam
25g/1oz chopped nuts

Drain the apricots and simmer for 20 minutes in 250ml/8fl oz (UK)/1C (US) of the apple juice until soft and most of the liquid is absorbed. Mash the apricots with a potato masher or put through a blender and place equal amounts into six dessert glasses. In a blender, mix half of the tofu with the rest of the ingredients except the nuts and then gradually add the remaining tofu. Blend until smooth. Pour the mixture on top of the apricots and chill. Before serving, sprinkle with the chopped nuts.

# CHAPTER 8

# Autumn

*Season of mists and mellow fruitfulness*
*Close bosom-friend of the maturing sun;*
*Conspiring with him how to load and bless*
*With fruit the vines that round the thatch-eaves run.*

JOHN KEATS

As summer drifts into late September, it gently begins to fade into amber-laced skies. And on the 23rd of the month autumn takes its rightful stand amongst its predecessors.

As with the spring equinox, autumn marks a time when darkness equals light, and day and night are equal. From here on, the nights draw in earlier and earlier, like a black velvet curtain closing in upon a golden stage. This continues until we reach the longest night of the year, on 21 December.

Autumn is the season of maturity and harvest, the early part exhibiting the results of summer's climax. For nature, the next few months are a most busy time. Small mammals gather and store the produce of past weeks, birds take flight, and plant life, too, braces itself for the coming winter frosts.

In the human world, it's also a time to make provisions. Practically speaking, this means swapping our sandals and shorts for warmer garb and planning preparations for the autumn era. On other levels as well, both mentally and spiritually, we can reassess our present situation. Summer projects, if favourable, are best brought to a head, tying up the ends of any unfinished business. We can then collect our thoughts and ideas and begin to direct our energies inwardly.

Autumn is an excellent time to commence or restart intellectual pursuits. Reading, writing or maybe enrolling on a new course of study all seem appropriate autumn-like things to do. And with most teaching faculties reopening after the summer break, the brain-storming world is our oyster.

Besides keeping our mind stimulated, we should continue to participate in some form of exercise programme, possibly slowly moving away from outdoor activities and choosing to join a gym or sports centre. Raising the heart rate for a period of 20 minutes or more, three to four times a week, has shown to reduce the risk of heart disease, cancer, high blood pressure, diabetes, obesity, depression and a swarm of other existing dispositions.

## AN AUTUMN DIET

When summer links with autumn, we can take advantage of the last of the sun's offspring in the form of a variety of local fruits. See, for instance, the delicious recipe for sugar-free blackberry jam on page 146. Apples, pears, grapes and an assortment of berries are wildly abundant at this time of year, and make the ideal ingredients for a final end-of-summer cleanse. The elimination period is best undertaken around the time of the equinox – or certainly no later than mid-October. This sets us up for a fuller dietary discipline, in anticipation for the advancing colder days.

By November, fruit consumption should be greatly reduced, one or two pieces of the late-comers (usually apples and pears), being adequate each day. Any extra pickings can be transformed into home-made, sugarless jam and the leftovers, particularly berries, can be frozen and used at a later date.

Although this book has been built around seasonal eating, there's nothing wrong in preserving specific foods, as long as it is done without the aid of artificial preservatives and other unnatural agents. Just as some countryside creatures bury acorns and nuts as food to fall back on, naturally conserving out-of-season produce is a commonsense means of getting through the cold. This doesn't mean to say that saving everything is the right way to go. But fruits such as raspberries and blackberries and many summer herbs do preserve rather well, adding a ray of sunshine to the winter dinner plate.

To naturally preserve fresh herbs, lay them out on a large tray and leave in a warm, dry but airy place. They also need to be kept away from direct sunlight. A porch, shady corner of the kitchen, airing cupboard or garden shed are all suitable locations. Under good conditions, herbs usually take about four to five days to dry. Before removing them from their stems, be sure they are not too damp, as they will turn mouldy if bottled too early. At the same time, do not leave them so long that they become powdery and over-dry. Once reaped, store them in airtight containers, preferably made from coloured glass.

## HEALTHFUL HARVEST

Following the grand autumn harvest, we start to see other, slightly heavier crops emerging from the ground. Starchy pumpkins and squash, coarse dark greens and thick root vegetables gradually replace the summery leaves and stems. Sea vegetables also make an excellent autumn supplement, adding copious minerals to the diet.

If we wish to keep our health throughout the autumn we must remodel our style of eating and aim for a more concentrated regime. This means cutting back on salads and sprouted grains and seeds and opting for a larger percentage of cooked pulses, vegetables and grains.

For those living in areas that get extremely cold some animal foods may be included, as they can when they appeal to you. Free-range eggs and goat's milk produce are the least offensive of these, and do not overburden the system as flesh foods do.

Those wishing to stick to a pure vegetarian regime can obtain extra nourishment by increasing the amount of tofu, tempeh and seitan in the diet. Although tofu has a potentially cooling effect upon the body, if cooked in the correct fashion, with the right blend of seasoning (garlic and ginger are heat-producing), its energy can be transformed into one that resumes warmth.

**The squash family**

Along with the nostalgia of the autumn harvest comes the delights of the vibrant, thick-skinned squash family, bursting at the seams with prospective goodness.

Squash can be divided into two categories: summer squash, which includes courgettes (zucchini) and crookneck, and winter squash, such as acorn, butternut, spaghetti, gem and, last but not least, pumpkin. In this chapter we shall concentrate on the winter selection.

Reckoned to be one of the earliest of cultivated vegetables, the pumpkin originated on the continent of America. It was later introduced to Britain, around the sixteenth century, where it became a cheap and cheerful energy food. However in the last century or so its popularity has waned, providing little more than a party piece for October's Hallowe'en.

To revive the assets of this exotic-looking vegetable, here's a résumé of its interesting innards.

The pumpkin, like its relatives, is an excellent source of fibre and good-quality carbohydrate, its bright orange skin giving obvious signs of beta-carotene. This is entwined with moderate amounts of calcium and potassium, and a shuffle of B vitamins and vitamin C.

Being delicately flavoured, pumpkin flesh can be used in sweet

*Figure 14, Winter squash*

| Squash | Shape/size | Rind colour | Extra information |
|--------|-----------|-------------|-------------------|
| Acorn | ribbed, pumpkin-style | green | |
| Butternut | club-shaped | creamy yellow | sweet, nutty flavour |
| Gem | small and round like a tennis ball | green | |
| Spaghetti | cylindrical formation | yellow | stringy spaghetti-ish flesh |
| Kabocha | similar to a medium pumpkin | blue-green | sweetest of all squash |

and savoury dishes alike, and makes a pleasant change to potatoes or grain. As for storage, winter squash keep exceedingly well and maintain their edibility for many weeks. You can even use them for first aid, applying the flesh to burns and scalds.

Why not hunt down the many varieties of squash that can be chanced upon? Figure 14 lists some of the most popular kinds and their conspicuous features.

*Squash cooking suggestions*

These weird and wonderful specimens can be prepared in a variety of ways.

The simplest method of cooking squash is to cut it in half, remove the seeds, coat the flesh with a teaspoon or so of olive oil, season with black pepper and bake face down on a moderate heat until tender. This usually takes about 30–45 minutes. It can then be eaten on its own or the hollows can be filled with an already-made casserole or vegetable sauce – a real treat on cool, crisp evenings.

Squash can also be steamed or sautéed, softening within 10 to 15 minutes. To prepare, cut into wedges, remove seeds, peel off the outer skin and chop into large chunks. Once cooked, it can either be puréed or added to stews and other savouries. Squash purée is a splendid ingredient and makes a delicious base for sauces and soups. Its naturally sweet flavour also makes it an ideal filler for muffins and cakes, helping to reduce the need for other, less wholesome, sweeteners.

On removing the seeds from pumpkins, don't throw them away. Roast them in a lightly heated oven and then toast them in a dry, thick-bottomed skillet for a few minutes. They can then be stored in a sealed container and will stay fresh for several months.

**Overlooked autumn vegetables**

We all know the carrots and potatoes of this world, but there are other interesting vegetables just waiting to hit the spotlight. To broaden the autumn horizon, here are five less popular plants in need of some special attention.

## Celeriac

Celeriac is a large, cream-coloured root with a rough, knobbly skin. Subtly scented of celery, it forms part of the parsley family and provides us with potassium, calcium and vitamin C.

Celeriac can be peeled and cooked in the same way as carrots or rutabaga (swede), either steamed or boiled in minimal liquid. It can also be grated and added to root salads or coleslaw.

## Fennel

Licorice lovers can delight in this attractive, aniseed-flavoured bulb. Fennel is a compact vegetable with tightly compressed leaves and protruding branches. Its medicinal properties date back to ancient times, and today it's still used as a food remedy. Like fennel tea, the root helps conquer intestinal gas and aids digestion.

Fennel is prepared by trimming away its feathery stems and slicing and steaming the root. Alternatively, it can be finely slivered and mixed into salads and stir-fries. The fronds can be reserved as a garnish or seasoning.

## Jerusalem artichokes

The Jerusalem variety of artichoke looks like a small knotty potato, and can be treated in much the same way. It contains decent quantities of calcium and iron and encompasses the polysaccharide inulin, a non-usable carbohydrate, that aids blood-sugar balance and alleviates constipation.

Jerusalem artichokes can be peeled and steamed or roasted, used instead of potatoes in potato salad or – once in a blue moon – fried like chips.

*Kohlrabi*

Kohlrabi belongs to the cabbage family and offers another cool-season filler to add to the cooking pot. The vegetable can appear white, light green or pale purple in colour, with a round base and shooting, leafy stems. Flavour-wise, kohlrabi is similar to a mild turnip, the smaller ones being the most tasteful. Kohlrabi juice can also be drunk to ease nosebleeds and bleeding of the colon.

Kohlrabi is best steamed, added to soups or grated, uncooked for salads.

*Marrow*

Native to South America, it's believed that this oft-neglected member of the squash family – the marrow – first hit British shores in the 1800s, where it became a common garden vegetable. Today, although its appeal has dwindled, it provides yet another casserole celebrity, yielding small amounts of potassium, calcium and vitamins A and C.

To serve marrow, slice and deseed it and then steam or gently fry. It's also a good stuffing vegetable and can be filled and baked with a mix and match of ingredients.

**Sea treasures**

Sea vegetables are a real catch, brimming with flavour and subsistence. Not many people know it, but these unusual edibles contain more minerals than any other plant. They also possess up to 50 per cent protein, a compilation of vitamins and very little fat. Vegans and vegetarians should regularly include this food group in their diet. It's a good source of iron and vitamin $B_{12}$ and some varieties contain more calcium than milk. A significant amount of iodine is also present, vital for the proper functioning of the thyroid gland.

Another outstanding feature of seaweed is a fibre molecule known as alginic acid. This substance has the ability to bind in the body with heavy metals such as cadmium, mercury and lead and carry them out of the alimentary tract. Some types of seaweed, namely kombu and hijiki, also contain sodium alginate, a hydrophilic colloidal component, that chelates radioactive material (absorbed through X-rays, television and other low-level radiation emitters) and removes it from the system.

Sounds like a perfect food? Well, the only downside to these mainly Japanese jewels is associated with the waters from which they come.[1] With widespread pollution in coastal areas, it's important to know where commercial supplies of seaweed are harvested. Fortunately, the major importers in the West maintain that all their supplies have been taken from clean sites and are routinely tested at independent laboratories.

Because fresh sea vegetables tend to spoil quickly, they're most often sold in their dried, long-life state. To allow for palate adjustment they are best introduced gradually into the diet, and then savoured in small servings three or four times a week. Being very concentrated, 10g/⅓oz (in its dry state) per meal is sufficient – and once rehydrated, a little goes a long way.

Let's now consider seven of these wholesome wonders (the description given for each one is of its appearance in its dried state, rather than in its original form, when taken from the sea).

*Agar-agar*

Looks like: Fine transparent flakes or powder.
Flavour: Neutral/bland.
Originates from: Japan.
How to use it: Agar-agar is sold as a vegetarian gelling agent – in place of and far superior to gelatine. Because of its blandness, agar-agar can be used in recipes that are either sweet or savoury in nature, such as jellies or aspics. To achieve great tasting jelly, mix 3 heaped tbsp of agar-agar flakes or powder into 600ml/2fl oz (UK)/2¾C (US) of boiling fruit juice and simmer for 3 minutes until all the seaweed has dissolved. Pour the liquid into a mould and leave to cool. It will set without refrigeration.

Entertaining extras: Agar-agar is calorie-free.

*Arame*

Looks like: Thin, black threadlike strands.
Flavour: Mild.
Originates from: Japan.
How to use it: Rehydrate it by soaking in water for five minutes, whereupon it will double in size. It can then be combined with salads or steamed, sautéed or added to soups. Arame softens within minutes and is delicious eaten with noodles, rice, tofu or vegetables.
Entertaining extras: Because arame is relatively mild in taste, it's a good one to try for those who are new to this food collection. As a folk remedy, arame is known as a treatment for female reproductive disorders.

*Dulse*

Looks like: Purple-red flat fronds (leaves).
Flavour: Peppery/spice-like.
Originates from: Eastern Canada.
How to use it: Wash it well before use, as dulse, unlike many of the other sea plants, has undergone little in the way of primary processing procedures. It may therefore harbour bits of debris and seashell.
  Dulse can be dry-roasted over an open flame (in which case do not soak) and then eaten as a snack, or ground down in a nut grinder to produce a healthy salt substitute. Alternatively, soak for 10 minutes, then steam, sauté or add to casseroles during the final five minutes of cooking. Also use to pep up soups, pâtés, vegetable burgers and grains.
Entertaining extras: Dulse is considered to be the most iron-rich of all seaweeds and also supplies good amounts of potassium, magnesium and iodine. Therapeutically, eaten in small amounts dulse is an effective remedy for sea sickness.

## Hijiki

Looks like: Arame, only the strands are slightly thicker and more wiry.
Flavour: Strong.
Originates from: Japan.
How to use it: Soak it for 15 minutes then sauté until soft, or employ in the same way as arame. As hijiki expands almost fivefold when hydrated, only very small amounts are necessary.
Entertaining extras: Once ingested, hijiki swells like fibre in the colon, helping to regulate blood-sugar levels and normalize the not-so-meritable fats. It also has an effect as a mild diuretic and due to its high concentration of calcium is a good bone-builder and adds lustre to the hair.

## Kombu

Looks like: Broad, dark, wrinkled strips.
Flavour: Rich.
Originates from: Japan.[2]
How to use it: With a pair of scissors, cut it into convenient pieces and soak for 30 minutes. Then add to home-made soups, beans or slow-cooking casseroles. Due to the presence of glutamic acid, a naturally occurring version of monosodium glutamate (MSG), kombu can also be used as a flavour enhancer, and incorporated into stocks and broths.
Entertaining extras: Kombu is rich in a number of minerals, greatly enhancing the nutrient value of all meals cooked with it. It also improves the flavour and digestibility of other food (especially those high in protein) during the simmering process.

Kombu's nourishing combination means that when included regularly in the diet it can help ease the pains of arthritis and the symptoms of goitre, high blood pressure, rheumatism, enlarged prostate and anaemia.

## Nori

Looks like: Thin, flat dark sheets.
Flavour: 'Fishy'.
Originates from: Japan.
How to use it: Nori sheets can be crisped up by passing over a medium flame, changing the colour from black to bright green. Nori sheets can also be purchased already toasted (sushi nori). Either cut it into fine strips or crumble it over soups and savouries. Another popular method of use is to treat each sheet as a base for sandwiching grains and twirl them into sushi rolls.
Entertaining extras: Nori contains as much protein as meat and eggs and matches the carrot in its content of beta-carotene. It's also the most easily digested of all sea vegetables, aiding the dissolution of fats and the breakdown of cholesterol.

*Figure 15, Some of the nutritional values of seaweed, compared to meat and milk*

| Food | Protein (g) | Fat (g) | Potassium (mgs per 100g) | Calcium (mgs) | Iron (mgs) |
|---|---|---|---|---|---|
| agar-agar | 2.3 | 0.1 | N/A | 400 | 5 |
| arame | 12.1 | 1.3 | 3,860 | 1,170 | 12 |
| dulse | 25 | 3.2 | 8,060 | 296 | 150 |
| hijiki | 5.6 | 0.8 | 14,700 | 1,400 | 29 |
| kombu | 7.3 | 1.1 | 5,800 | 800 | 15 |
| nori | 35 | 0.7 | N/A | 470 | 23 |
| wakame | 12.7 | 1.5 | 6,800 | 1,300 | 13 |
| cow's milk | 3.5 | 3.5 | 66 | 118 | trace |
| steak | 19.4 | 17.5 | 319 | 5.7 | 1.87 |

Source: USDA and Japan Nutritionist Association Foods tables and the Standard Tables of Food Composition in Japan.

*Wakame*

Looks like: Kombu, in its dried state, but once soaked resembles leafy greens.
Flavour: Light.
Originates from: Japan.
How to use it: Rehydrate it in water for five minutes, then add to soups or steam it with other vegetables. It can also be sautéed or simmered and mixed with grains and noodles or used as a filling for sandwiches. As a special treat, deep-fry and eat as sea chips.
Entertaining extras: Like kombu, wakame helps tenderize hard-to-digest food by softening tough fibres. It's also an all-round sovereign of nutrition.

## AUTUMN ELIMINATION

Unlike spring, where a more grain-based cleanse is seasonable, the fruits of autumn are unrestricted. As previously mentioned, early autumn's assemblance of fruited fixtures provides a perfect opportunity for a pre-winter cleanse. This can take the form of a three-day fruit fast or longer if need be. Mono-diets, such as grazing on grapes, have proved to be a worthy way of cleaning the whole system and many have cast themselves of some of the most dreaded diseases by way of this discipline.

I once observed a friend who ate nothing but grapes through the month of September. Admittedly, she had no major complications to deal with, only niggling nuisances such as the gradual materialization of a fleshy tyre around her abdomen and a few skin blemishes. During the four weeks, only grapes, grape juice and water passed her lips. She experienced no hunger pangs or cravings and her energy levels remained high. By the end of the month she looked 10 years younger, was 10lbs lighter and scored 10 out of 10 for immaculately glowing skin.

Of course a fruit fast, however satisfactory for some, is not suited to everyone's needs. Those with *Candida albicans* overgrowth or blood-sugar problems, or who become easily ungrounded, are advised to use other tools towards purification. The spring cleansing programme outlined on page 68, for example, can be repeated instead and offers a less 'yin' alternative.

## Skin brushing

To enhance the passage of toxins from the system, skin brushing should become part and parcel of the daily routine.

The skin (although not thought of as such) is the largest organ of the body. Besides helping to keep us in one piece, it assists in the exit of waste. If the skin becomes blocked with dead cells and debris, toxins from within will be unable to escape productively, putting a greater burden on other routes of elimination. If these organs become overworked, an accumulation of rubbish can build up inside, exacerbating an already 'muddy' condition.

Skin brushing requires a pure vegetable-bristle brush. Similar synthetics are not advised.

The best time to brush the skin is just before taking a bath or shower, when the skin is still dry. Begin by brushing the extremities; up the hands, arms, feet and legs and in towards the centre of the body, moving the brush in brisk stroking movements. Then brush down the back and chest and back up the abdomen towards the thorax again.

At first, the brush may feel quite rough on the skin, but this sensitivity will quickly pass. The face area, being very delicate, should not be included in the routine.

By regularly brushing the body, several modes of action can be accomplished:

- Blood circulation is improved.
- The lymphatic system is stimulated.
- Immunity is enhanced.
- Impurities are removed.
- Skin becomes softer.
- There is an increased all-over vigour.
- Cellulite is encouraged to disperse.

# AUTUMN COOKING TECHNIQUES

Parallel to spring, autumn cooking calls for receptiveness and versatility, with a swing from a raw venture to a more cooked/macrobiotic phase. We no longer require ladles of cooling elements, accentuated by salads, but need to gather in warmth from the application of heat.

Now although cooking fresh food is often shunned in the world of nutrition, if prepared in the correct manner high-quality nourishment can be maintained. Choose from waterless simmering, steaming and grilling, to stir-frying, sautéing and the big bake. Uncooked foods can accompany main meals in this season.

Sautéing food in a little oil, especially flavour-enhancing garlic, onions and spices, can be used as a base for the art of soup-making or in the preparation of autumn-fit stews, casseroles and hot-pots. This method initially brings out the zest of certain vegetables, whilst the oil adds a thicker, creamier texture to the dish.

With the need to assign more time to the kitchen in the chillier months of the calendar, don't be tempted to compromise quality for convenience with the use of a microwave. Cooking food, or even reheating it, in a microwave oven is the most unnatural way of assembling a meal. Whilst fire (as in a gas cooker) heats food by friction, microwaves do the job by changing the polarity of the food's atoms thousands of times per second, thus mutating the normal electromagnetic field.

Fats and vitamin content are affected, and the life force, especially in vegetables, is completely destroyed. It has also been noted that protein molecules in food are transformed into unstable units. Microwave ovens may leak radiation whilst in operation too. Eating food that has been cooked in this way, on a regular basis, will eventually have a negative rebound on the tissues of the body, leading to weakness and nervous disorders. I advise everyone, especially those who are unwell, to steer well clear of microwave ovens – whether for cooking or reheating purposes.

Just as it's important to produce and eat healthy, nutritious meals, the cook must also carry a healthy disposition.

Someone who prepares food while tired, upset, angry or in a pessimistic frame of mind will offload these qualities and pass on the subtle negative energies to anyone who eats the food.

It's therefore wise to take a few minutes out before entering the kitchen, to unwind and relax and quieten the mind. During the cooking process, cheerful, elevating background music can be played to help raise the consciousness; keeping the kitchen area clean and tidy will also help.

## AUTUMN REVIEW

1 Devote some time to a three-day (or longer) fruit fast.
2 Begin to eat less raw food and more cooked.
3 Become familiar with the squash clan and other less popular vegetables.
4 Experiment with seaweeds.
5 Bring unfinished projects to a close.
6 Enrol on a new course of study.
7 Join a fitness centre.

To conclude our visit to autumn, here's a shopping guide to the fresh produce in season. It also includes a variety of dried wholefoods, which although aren't distinct to autumn are essential store-cupboard provisions.

*Figure 16, Fresh foods in autumn*

| Nuts | Grains | Seeds |
| --- | --- | --- |
| almonds | amaranth | hemp |
| Brazil nuts | barley | linseed |
| cashew nuts | buckwheat | pumpkin |
| chestnuts | bulgar wheat | sesame |
| hazelnuts | maize | sunflower |
| macadamia nuts | millet | |
| peanuts | oats | |
| pecans | quinoa | |
| pine nuts | rice | |
| pistachios | wheat | |
| walnuts | wild rice | |

*Figure 16, Fresh foods in autumn* (cont.)

| Vegetables | Fruit | Herbs | Beans/Pulses |
|---|---|---|---|
| aubergines or eggplants | apples | bay leaf | adzuki |
| broccoli | blueberries | marjoram | black turtle |
| carrots | blackberries | parsley | black-eyed |
| celeriac | blackcurrants | sage | borlotti |
| celery | cranberries | rosemary | broad |
| chard | damsons | tarragon | cannellini |
| chicory | gooseberries | thyme | chickpeas |
| Chinese leaves | grapes | | field |
| courgettes | loganberries | | flageolet |
| cress | pears | | haricot |
| cucumbers | plums | | mung |
| fennel | raspberries | | pinto |
| garlic | rhubarb | | red kidney |
| horseradish | | | soya |
| Jerusalem artichokes | | | lentils |
| kale | | | split peas |
| kohlrabi | | | |
| leeks | | | |
| lettuces | | | |
| marrows | | | |
| mushrooms | | | |
| mooli | | | |
| onions | | | |
| peas | | | |
| potatoes | | | |
| swedes or rutabagas | | | |
| sweetcorn | | | |
| tomatoes | | | |
| turnips | | | |
| watercress | | | |
| winter squash | | | |

# RECIPES FOR AUTUMN

## Tofu, Runner Bean and Quinoa Salad
*Serves 6*

INGREDIENTS
200g/7oz quinoa
¼tsp (UK)/¼tsp(US) vegetable bouillon
200/7oz runner beans, trimmed and finely chopped
4tbsp untoasted sesame oil
200g/7oz leeks, trimmed and chopped
1 clove of garlic, peeled and crushed
200g/7oz marinated or smoked tofu, cubed
2 tomatoes, chopped
100g/4oz chicory, finely shredded
1tsp (UK)/1tsp (US) tamari
1tsp tabasco
1tsp lemon juice
½tsp (UK)/½tsp (US) toasted sesame oil

Wash the quinoa well and simmer with the vegetable bouillon in twice the volume of boiling water for 12–15 minutes or until all the liquid has been absorbed and the grain is soft. Set aside.

In a separate saucepan, steam the runner beans for 10 minutes and set aside. Then put the untoasted sesame oil into another pan and sauté the leeks, garlic and tofu, stirring frequently, until the leeks are cooked.

Finally, place the cooked contents from all three saucepans into a bowl, add the tomatoes, chicory, tamari, tabasco, lemon juice and toasted sesame oil and mix.

## Chicory, Chard and Tomato Salad
*Serves 6*

INGREDIENTS
200g/7oz fine green beans, trimmed
50g/2oz chicory, finely chopped
50g/2oz Swiss chard, finely chopped
450g/1lb tomatoes, chopped
50g/2oz unsalted peanuts
Dressing
4tbsp (UK)/⅓C (US) plain goat's or soya yoghurt
1 clove of garlic, trimmed and crushed
1 heaped tsp paprika
¼ heaped tsp freeze-dried coriander leaf

Steam the beans for 12 minutes until soft, place them in a bowl and leave to cool. Add chicory, Swiss chard, tomatoes, peanuts and dressing ingredients and gently combine. Chill until ready to serve.

## Tofu, Sea Vegetables and Sun-dried Tomato Sandwich
*Serves 6*

INGREDIENTS
150g/5oz carrots, peeled and grated
3tbsp (UK)/¼C (US) tofu mayonnaise
1 loaf of 100 per cent wholemeal flour or spelt flour bread
150g/5oz hummus
100g/4oz mixed lettuce leaves
8 strips of wakame, rehydrated
250g/9oz marinated tofu, sliced
15g/½oz sun-dried tomatoes, rehydrated

Mix the carrots and tofu mayonnaise together and set aside.

Slice the bread into twelve slices, spreading each one with a thin layer of hummus. Then on six of the slices generously layer in order lettuce, the carrot mixture, wakame, tofu and tomatoes. Place the remaining slices of bread on top of each sandwich and serve.

## Buckwheat Harvest Stir-Fry
*Serves 4*

INGREDIENTS
225g/8oz shallots, peeled and sliced
2 cloves of garlic, peeled and crushed
1 red pepper, deseeded and sliced
1 green pepper, deseeded and sliced
1 yellow pepper, deseeded and sliced
2tbsp (UK)/3tbsp (US) sesame oil
200g/7oz runner beans, trimmed and chopped into small pieces
1tbsp (UK)/1½tbsp (US) tamari
250g/9oz buckwheat soba[3]
100g/4oz sunflower seeds
100ml/4fl oz (UK)/½C (US) water
sea salt and black pepper

In a wok or large skillet sauté the shallots, garlic and peppers in the sesame oil for a few minutes, then add the runner beans and allow to simmer for a further 12 minutes. Add the tamari, wait until most of it has been absorbed and set aside.

Whilst the stir-fry ingredients are cooking bring a saucepan of water to boil, add the buckwheat soba and simmer for 10 minutes until soft. Drain well and place in a bowl.

In a nut grinder, grind down the sunflower seeds, then mix with the water to form a smooth paste. Season and gently blend it into the buckwheat.

Finally, serve the stir-fried vegetables on top of the buckwheat.

## Fried Polenta with Aubergine or Eggplant in a Rich Walnut Sauce
*Serves 8*

INGREDIENTS
1 medium aubergine or eggplant, trimmed
sea salt
150ml/¼ pint (UK)/⅔C (US) olive oil
250g/9oz polenta
700ml/1¼ pints (UK)/3C (US) water
1 onion, peeled and chopped
2 cloves of garlic, peeled and crushed
1 red pepper, deseeded and finely sliced
1 heaped tsp paprika
One 400g/14oz tin of chopped tomatoes
1 carrot, peeled and grated
1tsp (UK)/1tsp (US) vegetable bouillon
3 heaped tbsp chopped fresh parsley
100g/4oz walnuts
200g/7oz goat's Cheddar or firm soya cheese

Cut the aubergine or eggplant into slices, sprinkle with sea salt and place on a paper towel for 30 minutes. Rinse off the salt, brush both sides with some of the olive oil and roast in a preheated oven on an oiled baking tray at 220°C/425°F/Gas 7 for 45 minutes. Set aside and leave the oven on.

Combine the polenta and water with a little sea salt in a saucepan, bring to the boil and simmer for 5 minutes, stirring occasionally. Place the cooked polenta into a mould (I use a spare plastic measuring cup) and leave to set.

Gently sauté the onion, garlic, red pepper and paprika in 2tbsps (UK)/3tbsp (US) of the olive oil. When the onions are transparent, add the tin of tomatoes and the carrot, vegetable bouillon and parsley and simmer for 15 minutes. Briefly dry-roast the walnuts in a skillet, then place them together with the prepared tomato sauce in a blender and whizz until smooth.

Remove the polenta from the mould (it should come out in one solid block), slice it into thin wedges and shallow-fry on both sides in the remaining olive oil. On a plate arrange the aubergine or eggplant on top of the fried polenta slices, pour on the tomato sauce and sprinkle with cheese. Serve immediately.

## Black Olive Tortilla
*Serves 4–6*

*A sustaining meal, simple and speedy to prepare. Serve with salad.*

450g/1lb potatoes, peeled and chopped into small pieces
100g/4oz pitted black olives
2 tomatoes, chopped
5 heaped tbsps chopped fresh flat-leaf parsley
1tbsp (UK)/1½tbsp (US) olive oil plus extra for oiling
2 cloves of garlic, peeled and crushed
1 onion, peeled and chopped
1 green pepper, deseeded and finely chopped
4 free-range eggs
1tbsp (UK)/1½tbsp (US) soya sauce
¼tsp (UK)/¼tsp (US) vegetable bouillon
sea salt and black pepper

Steam the potato pieces for 15 minutes until soft and place in a bowl. Add the olives, tomatoes and parsley and mix.

Place the olive oil in a saucepan and sauté the garlic, onion and green pepper for 5 minutes, adding them to the potato mixture once cooked.

In another bowl whisk the eggs, soya sauce, vegetable bouillon, sea salt and black pepper and pour on to the vegetables. Gently stir all the ingredients together.

Oil a 20cm/8in diameter flan or pie dish, pour and press the mixture in ensuring that it's even and bake in a preheated oven at 190°C/375°F/Gas 5 for 30 minutes.

## Spaghetti and Beans in Sweet and Sour Sauce
*Serves 4–6*

900g/2lb butternut squash (or other variety)
6tbsp (UK)/²/₃C (US) olive oil
100g/4oz pinto beans, soaked overnight
1 strip of kombu, rehydrated
a pinch of celery seeds
¼ heaped tsp cumin powder
200g/7oz carrots, peeled and cut into small sticks
100/4oz celery, finely chopped
200g/7oz kohlrabi, peeled and chopped
300ml/½ pint (UK)/1¼C (US) tomato or mixed vegetable juice
½tsp (UK)/½tsp (US) vegetable bouillon
1 onion, peeled and chopped
1 clove of garlic, peeled and crushed
1tbsp (UK)/1½tbsp (US) brown rice vinegar
1tbsp (UK)/1½tbsp (US) soya sauce
sea salt and black pepper
300g/11oz wholemeal, spelt or rice spaghetti

Cut the squash into quarters, remove and discard the seeds, coat the flesh with 2tbsp (UK)/3tbsp (US) of olive oil and bake face down in a preheated oven at 220°C/425°F/Gas 7 for 45–50 minutes, until soft. Once cooked, scoop out the flesh and mash it. Leave to one side.

Meanwhile, drain the beans, rinse and simmer in boiling water with the kombu for about 1 hour until soft, adding the celery seeds and cumin during the cooking process. Drain and set aside.

Place 2tbsp (UK)/3tbsp (US) of the olive oil in a saucepan, add the carrots, celery and the kohlrabi and sauté for 5 minutes. Add two-thirds of the tomato or mixed vegetable juice, the cooked pinto beans and the vegetable bouillon and simmer for 25–30 minutes.

In another saucepan, fry the onion and garlic in 2tbsp (UK)/3tbsp (US) of the olive oil for 5 minutes. Then add the mashed squash and the remaining tomato or mixed vegetable juice and continue to simmer for a few minutes. Finally, add the rice vinegar, soya sauce, sea salt and black pepper and stir.

Combine the squash mixture with the beans and vegetables and mix.

Boil the spaghetti according to the instructions on the packet and serve
with the sauce on top.


## Spicy Potato Rolls
*Makes 8*

INGREDIENTS
1.5kg/3½lbs potatoes, peeled and chopped
200g/7oz carrots, peeled and chopped
One 200g/7oz can of garden peas, drained
sea salt and black pepper
2 heaped tbsp mustard seeds
1tbsp (UK)/1½tbsp (US) unhydrogenated margarine (optional)
2 heaped tbsp mustard seeds
1tbsp (UK)/1½tbsp (US) olive oil
300g/11oz spelt flour, sieved
175ml/6fl oz (UK)/¾C (US) water

Steam the potatoes and carrots for 25 minutes until very soft. Add the
peas, sea salt, pepper and margarine (if using) and mash well ensuring
that there are no lumps. Gently fry the mustard seeds in the olive oil for
a few minutes and combine with the potato mixture.

In a bowl mix the spelt flour with the sea salt and the water, form into
a dough and divide into eight pieces. Roll out each piece with a rolling
pin into rounds each measuring about 20cm/8in across. In a dry skillet
or frying pan heat each side of the dough until well cooked. Place on a
plate. Divide the filling into eight, arrange the mixture along one side of
the bread and roll it up.

## Mexican Style Pumpkin
*Serves 4*

INGREDIENTS
2 medium-sized pumpkins
5tbsp (UK)/½C (US) olive oil
sea salt and black pepper
150g/5oz red kidney beans, soaked overnight
1 strip of kombu, rehydrated
1 clove of garlic, peeled and crushed
200g/7oz carrots, peeled and chopped
2 courgettes or zucchini, trimmed and chopped
75g/3oz baby corn, trimmed and chopped
One 400g/14oz can of chopped tomatoes
1 heaped tbsp paprika
½ heaped tsp mild chilli powder
1 fresh whole green chilli
1tbsp (UK)/1½tbsp (US) tamari

Drain and rinse the beans and simmer in boiling water with the kombu for 1 hour 30 minutes, until soft.

Meanwhile, cut the pumpkins in half, remove and discard the seeds and brush the flesh with a little of the olive oil. Season with sea salt and pepper and bake face down in a preheated oven at 220°C/425°F/Gas 7 for 50 minutes or until soft. Reserve.

After the beans have cooked for one hour, sauté the garlic, carrots, courgettes or zucchini and baby corn in the remaining olive oil for 5 minutes. Then add the tomatoes, paprika, chilli powder and whole green chilli and simmer for 20 minutes. Towards the end of the cooking time check the beans; when soft, drain them and add them with the tamari and mix. Remove the chilli and discard it, season the sauce and serve it on the baked pumpkin.

## Mixed Nut, Rice and Feta Parcels
*Makes 16 parcels*

INGREDIENTS
1 onion, peeled and chopped
2 medium courgettes or zucchini, trimmed and finely chopped
1tbsp (UK)/1½tbsp (US) olive oil and a little for oiling
225g/8oz long-grain brown rice
575ml/1 pint (UK)/2½C (US) tomato or mixed vegetable juice
400ml/14fl oz (UK)/⅔C (US) water
100g/4oz chopped mixed nuts
3 heaped tbsp toasted nori flakes
50g/2oz vegetarian feta cheese, grated
75g/1½lb frozen, ready-made vegetarian puff pastry, thawed and
at room temperature

In a large saucepan, sauté the onions and courgettes or zucchini in the
olive oil until the onions are transparent. Add the rice and stir for a
further few minutes. Then pour in the tomato or mixed vegetable juice
and simmer until all the liquid has been absorbed. Add water and
nuts and continue to simmer until the rice is soft. Total simmering time
should be about 50 minutes. Once cooked, stir in the nori flakes and feta
cheese and leave to stand for 10 minutes with the saucepan lid on. Turn
into a clean bowl and leave to cool.

Divide the pastry into 16 balls, rolling out each one to about
12cm/5in in diameter. When the rice mixture is cool, place 2 heaped
tbsp of the filling in the centre of each pastry piece and wrap them up
into small parcels.

Place them on an oiled baking tray and bake in a preheated oven at
205°C/400°F/Gas 6 for 45 minutes, until lightly golden.

## Split Pea and Potato Soup
*Serves 4*

INGREDIENTS
1 onion, peeled and chopped
100g/4oz celery, chopped
2 heaped tbsp dried sage
2tbsp (UK)/3tbsp (US) olive oil
225g/8oz green split peas, soaked overnight
250g/9oz potatoes, peeled and chopped
150g/5oz carrots, peeled and chopped
5 dried bay leaves
½ heaped tsp celery seeds
1 strip of kombu, rehydrated
1.5 litres/2½ pints (UK)/6¼C (US) water
1tbsp (UK)/1½tbsp (US) tamari
black pepper

In a large saucepan sauté the onion, celery and sage in the olive oil for 5 minutes. Drain and rinse the peas, and then add them to the saucepan together with the potatoes, carrots, bay leaves, celery seeds, kombu and water. Bring to the boil and simmer for 1 hour 15 minutes or until the peas are very soft. More water may be required during the cooking.

Remove and discard the bay leaves and kombu, season with tamari and black pepper and blend the soup in a liquidizer until smooth. Reheat and serve.

## Mixed Berry Trifle
*Serves 8*

100g/4oz crunchy, sugar-free granola
5 heaped tbsp sugarless mixed berry jam
300ml/½ pint (UK)/1¾C (US) raspberry or blackcurrant juice (use sugar-free concentrate and dilute down if necessary)
2 heaped tbsp agar-agar flakes
575ml/1 pint (UK)/2½C (US) of creamy vanilla soya milk
2 heaped tbsp cornflour
1tbsp (UK)/1½tbsp (US) natural red food colouring or beetroot juice
1tbsp (UK)/1½tbsp (US) natural raspberry flavour
1tbsp (UK)/1½tbsp (US) maize or brown rice syrup
575ml/1 pint (UK)/2½C (US) natural goat's or soya yoghurt
300g/11oz mixed berries

Mix the crunchy granola and sugar-free jam together and place in the bottom of a trifle dish.

Heat the fruit juice in a saucepan with the agar-agar flakes and simmer until the agar has dissolved. Pour on top of the granola mixture and leave to set.

Warm 500ml/16fl oz (UK)/2C (US) of the soya milk in a saucepan. In a bowl combine the remaining soya milk and the cornflour into a smooth paste and add to the saucepan, stirring all the time. Once thickened into a custard, take off the heat, mix in the red food colouring and the natural raspberry flavour and add to the trifle bowl. Leave to cool and set.

Stir the grain syrup into the yoghurt and pour over the top of the trifle; decorate with the berries and chill.

**Praline Crème Pears**
*Serves 6*

INGREDIENTS
300ml/½ pint (UK)/1¼C (US) apple or pear juice
6 pears, peeled, trimmed and sliced lengthways in half
275g/10oz plain firm tofu
3tbsp (UK)/¼C (US) maize or brown rice syrup
2 heaped tbsp hazelnut butter
1 heaped tsp carob powder
1tsp (UK)/1tsp (US) grain coffee substitute
1tbsp (UK)/1½tbsp (US) sunflower oil

Place about two-thirds of the fruit juice in a saucepan and simmer the pears for 5–10 minutes until soft and liquid has evaporated. Set aside and allow to cool.

To prepare the sauce, place the remaining fruit juice in a blender. Add the tofu and grain syrup and blend until smooth. Then add the hazelnut butter, carob powder, grain coffee substitute and sunflower oil and continue to blend. When all the ingredients are well combined, pour into a bowl and chill. Serve on top of the cooked pears.

**Blackberry Jam (sugar-free)**

INGREDIENTS
300ml/11fl oz apple or apple and blackcurrant concentrate
600g/1lb 5oz blackberries
3 tbsp kuzu root

In a saucepan bring the juice concentrate and blackberries to boil and simmer for 15 minutes.

Dissolve the kuzu in twice as much cold water and add to the fruit. Stir continuously for a few minutes whilst still on the heat, until mixture begins to thicken.

Once cool, store in an empty jam jar in the fridge and consume within two weeks.

# CHAPTER 9

# Winter

*In rigorous hours, when down the iron lane*
*The redbreast looks in vain*
*For hips and haws,*
*Lo, shining flowers upon my window pane*
*The silver pencil of the winter draws.*

*When all the snowy hill*
*And the bare woods are still;*
*When snipes are silent in the frozen bogs,*
*And all the garden garth is whelmed in mire,*
*Lo, by the hearth, the laughter of the logs –*
*More fair than roses, lo, the flowers of fire!*

ROBERT LOUIS STEVENSON

Autumn folds in on 21 December, time of the final biannual solstice, heralding winter as the season of dominance.

Winter is the term of nature's rest – in both the kingdom of animals and plants. Some creatures turn to hibernation, whilst others who prefer warmer climes have already left. Those which remain hide amongst the sleeping pastures, only venturing forth in a bid to survive.

Like our fellow beasts, we also need to slow the stride in the winter, relax more and be at peace. We should therefore spend less time out of the house, returning home after our day's deeds to continue our autumnal studies and be with family and friends.

Having earlier nights is harmonious in the season of winter; ideally, aim to hit the sack by 10 p.m. A short period of prayer or meditation before the lights are turned out will help quieten the mind and promote a good night's sleep.

Again, in the morning, we should choose to rise a little later than normal, just before or as the sun begins to dawn. Under-standably, in today's 'mad rush' society, this is often an impossible task, in which case it's doubly important not to have too many late nights. Nonetheless, this is not an excuse to laze around in bed or oversleep.

As for regular exercise, autumn's indoor activities can be extended, although slightly less aerobic vigour is necessary. Too much sweating can create needless energy loss and according to the Chinese allow microbes to invade the system via the open pores of the skin. If aerobic exercise is undertaken, don't wander out into the cold streets straight afterwards. First cool down, take a warm shower, dry thoroughly and wrap up warm.

Other forms of winter discipline can include yoga, t'ai chi and qigong, which demand less physical exertion, whilst keeping the mind and body in tip-top shape.

The winter solstice (the date of the longest night) and the weeks that follow can be a very susceptible period health-wise. Every year, many of us fall ill to the merciless common cold or worse still, the flu, having to spend several days at home tucked up in bed. The obvious reason for these untimely outbreaks is that most of us continue to burn the candle at both ends, ignoring winter's subtle commandments. Undoubtedly, the overindulgence of the Christmas festivities and the endless parties preceding the event don't help. Too much fat, sugar and alcohol consumed at this time can cause the body to become weak and congested; an accumulation of mucus and toxins is an ideal breeding ground for disease.

Another explanation for the rise in immune defectiveness is the routine handout of antibiotics, and amongst others the influenza vaccine. It must be realized that antibiotics do far more damage than good, pushing the symptoms of illness deeper into the system, instead of allowing them to surface and clear naturally.

As for the flu jab, injecting an alien substance into the body to protect it against a relatively mild virus that we may never get, seems pretty pointless. And with the possibility of strains changing from year to year, it's impossible to provide long-term protection by conventional means. The irony of it is that a shot of the flu vaccine is more likely to cause the flu than prevent it. Indeed, I have met many a person suffering from flu-like symptoms (possible inoculation side-effects) just after having a 'preventative' jab.

But the real worry with this vaccine – and all others when it boils down to it – is the long-term effects, especially in those who are immunized every year. Besides damaging the body's natural defence force, the foreign material that presents itself can remain within tissues for a long time, with the probability of causing far more virulent and chronic afflictions in the future.

The only true way of boosting the body's defence mechanism is to work alongside it, rather than against it. This we can do by nourishing ourselves with the right foods and herbs, avoiding the use of orthodox suppressive warfare, and where necessary augmenting our constitutions with appropriate nutritional supplements. To maintain optimum health throughout the winter, here are ten trouble-free ways to stay fighting fit.

1 Eat only wholefoods and fresh seasonal produce.
2 Exclude substances that destroy the body's nutrient store, such as sugar, tea, coffee, alcohol and cigarettes.
3 Eliminate foods that are highly acid- or mucus-forming. These include meat, dairy produce, refined foods and anything that's been fried.[1]
4 Add immune-amplifying herbs like garlic and ginger to meals and make it habitual to drink therapeutic teas. Ginger, rosehip, elderflower and peppermint are all noble chilly-season choices. Also look out for some excellent combination mixes specially designed with winter in mind.
5 Supplement the diet with extra nourishment in the way of a food-based algae product, for example, spirulina, chlorella or wild blue-green algae, or a combination of all three. Also take additional antioxidants, plus extra vitamin C. Select an antioxidant that contains at least 5–10mg of zinc and go for vitamin C in the form of magnesium ascorbate, a non-acidic, easily utilized preparation.

6 Indulge in warm, exhilarating baths, infused with aromatic essential oils. Lavender, lemon and teatree are worthy anti-cold remedies and serve a multitude of other purposes at the same time. Regular skin brushing also aids immunity by stimulating the lymphatics and eliminatory process.

7 Ensure frequent exercise, even if this only entails taking a brisk 20-minute walk twice daily.

8 Before going out, dress with plenty of layers – if necessary wearing a hat, gloves and scarf. Avoid the damp and draughts.

9 Take life at a steady pace, shirk stressful situations and allow time for work, rest and play.

10 Remain positive, cheerful and enthusiastic and enjoy the uniqueness that winter has to share.

*The inner voice*

If we do all the right things yet still succumb, we should know there is a good reason, and pay particular attention to what our body is trying to communicate. It may be that we genuinely need to take a rest, or allow ourselves time to dwell on a personal issue. In such cases, it's important to take some time out, go deep within and recuperate.

For those of us who live in a temperate climate, winter can often prove to be quite a hike. What with grey, barren days and long, bitter nights, even the jolliest of people may at points lose their smile.

But feeling down in the dumps at this time of year is far from being just in the mind. Research has confirmed that a lack of exposure to natural sunlight can alter the body's daily rhythms, causing us to encounter depression – from mild to severe.

To explain what happens in simple terms: when sunlight enters the eyes, it triggers the release of neurotransmitters (chemical nerve messengers) produced in the brain, and one of these is serotonin, the happiness enhancer. When the level of light declines, as it does in the winter, the deliverance of this 'feel-good' factor plummets – along with our moods. In addition to this, the hormone melatonin, which balances our sleep/wake cycle, is also disturbed, prompting us to experience the ascendance of doom and gloom.

The 'winter doldrums' is now a recognized condition, aptly named SAD (Seasonal Affective Disorder). Fortunately, this cold-season phenomenon can be efficiently overcome, responding remarkably well to the missing link – light. Sufferers undergo phototherapy, which involves exposing the eyes to a full-spectrum light. Light boxes which give out natural rays can also be installed in the home and left on for a couple of hours a day. To prevent symptoms from setting in, it's a good idea to commence the treatment from early October and continue right through to spring. Other ways to lighten up include:

- Get out in the open during the day, for a brief meander. Take a wander through the countryside or nearby park. However overcast it may seem, some light will always filter through.
- Replace artificial-light bulbs with daylight bulbs, which offer a more realistic lighting system.
- Eat plenty of vegetables, storers of condensed sunlight, and foods that are rich in complex carbohydrates, which boost serotonin levels.
- Brighten up the living space with mirrors and hanging crystals, which help reflect light.
- Exercise. Aerobic movement activates the production of brain chemicals that increase self-esteem and encourage a positive outlook.

## THE WINTER DIET

Winter eating habits follow on from the autumn table, with brilliant displays of edible roots, bright coloured pumpkins, cabbages, broccoli, Brussels sprouts and uncracked Christmassy nuts. Root vegetables such as carrots, parsnips, turnips, swede or rutabaga, onions and potatoes are superb for all winter dishes –

from the invention of simple soups and stews to flamboyant bisques and bakes. Legumes and grains also make up a large percentage of the winter diet and can be eaten together for good-quality protein and fuel. Grains should be rotated regularly, so as not to overeat one particular kind. Buckwheat and oats, the most heat-producing of cereals, are good winter selections.

As with the months gone by, continue to include other sources of vegetable protein on a daily basis – and if yearned for, free-range eggs, goat's milk and its by-products.

Fruit is highly limited in the winter weeks, with most temperate locations having only the last of the apples and pears to tell the tale. Fortunately, these store rather well in the refrigerator and provide fabulous fillings for pies and crumbles. Frozen berries that have been saved from the autumn harvest can also be improvised here. Cooking this food sector is advantageous in the winter, as it's likely to be rather cooling for the body in its raw state.

Dried fruit can also be eaten.

Most vegetables are best cooked in some way during the cold spell, so that their cooling properties are transformed into warming ones. Typical winter roots turn out far more palatable when soft and can be jazzed up with fresh winter herbs such as sage and rosemary. Salad vegetables can be eaten raw as a starter or side dish, instead of as a main course, and will attach that bit of freshness and vital vitamin C to the winter regime.

Just because it's cold outside, doesn't mean that we should cut down on our water intake. With electric or gas heating facilities installed in most homes, the effects of this constant energy can be very drying, causing our skin to wither and bodies to dehydrate. It might be a good idea to humidify the environment by placing a bucket of water near the radiator, and when possible to leave windows slightly ajar. This goes for air-conditioned offices too. As well as adequate water supplies, herbal teas can be sipped throughout the day, aiding winter body balance.

Throughout the winter there's often a tendency to eat more than usual. To a certain extent it's honest to say that on icy-cold days, we may need a few additional calories to keep us warm. But because we are likely to become less active, we must try not to eat more than we can burn.

Trading in out-of-season produce and items high in sugar and fat for locally grown, properly cooked food will certainly provide us with increased sustenance and prevent that feeling of emptiness inside. A good breakfast consisting of slow-releasing carbohydrates such as millet porridge or brown-rice pudding will keep us well stocked up until midday. Midday and evening meals should always be packed with plenty of vegetables and a good plant-based protein savoury to complement.

Thereafter we must learn to balance what we take in with our energy expenditure, so that by spring we won't have to work too hard at breaking down surplus storage.

**Roots to good health**

Roots are the predominant type of vegetable to flourish during the winter, so we shall now delve a little deeper into some rootful revelations.

Root vegetables (in which I include tubers and bulbs as well) are without doubt the most sustaining of all vegetables, helping us take on the harsh winter weather that they themselves have thrived in. Unlike most summery crops, roots grow downwards from the seed into the soil, absorbing the goodness from the earth and producing a sweeter, denser vegetable. Some root vegetables grow all year round, but the trend is more towards winter and spring. Root crops are especially suited to the winter because they store well and make excellent cold-season dishes.

Roots are rich in complex carbohydrates and therefore require slightly more digesting than other vegetable varieties. As a result, they go down better when cooked, which also enhances their warming qualities. Roots can be steamed, roasted, added to soups and savouries of all kinds, or softened and mashed, as we do with that popular species, the potato. When grated, many of them can be tolerated raw and eaten as salad.

Most root vegetables store very well for reasonable lengths of

*Figure 17, Common winter vegetables*

| Roots | Tubers | Bulbs |
|---|---|---|
| Beetroot | Jerusalem artichoke | Fennel |
| Carrot | Potato | Garlic |
| Celeriac | Sweet potato | Leeks |
| Parsnip | | Onion |
| Swede or rutabaga | | |
| Radish | | |
| Turnip | | |

time, and if kept in a cool, well-ventilated area, do not need to be refrigerated.

## Special roots

Two special roots that are used more for their intense flavours than as fillers, are garlic and ginger – typical ancient bestsellers. Apart from their culinary purposes, both are renowned for their many healing perks, some of which we will now take a look at.

### Garlic

This pungent bulb has a wonderful reputation, requiring a complete book of its own to reveal its true identity. I will do my best to disclose its goodness in this limited space.

First of all, garlic is an anti-congestor, clearing away excess mucus from the throat and respiratory tract. It also possesses antimicrobial attributes – intimidating bacteria, fungus and worms – and has been noted to help lower high blood pressure and the dangerous LDL (low-density lipoprotein) fats. On top of this, garlic inhibits abnormal blood clotting and purifies the blood – making it a fighting food for a healthy heart.

Much of garlic's positive features are linked closely to its rich combination of sulphur-containing compounds, some of which give this bulb its characteristic odour. Other interesting factors include the cancer inhibitors selenium and germanium and the amino acid cysteine.

Whilst the raw stuff is often backed by converted garlic fans, too much (besides being unsociable), may cause a burning sensation in the mouth and digestive tract. Consequently it should only be taken this way in small amounts. In traditional Chinese medicine garlic is better when briefly cooked, whereupon the compound that causes aggravation is dispersed, leaving much of the goodness still active.

### Ginger

Ginger root, although a hot-climate edible, can be thought of more as a medicine than a food, which allows us to introduce it into our seasonal eating plan. Like garlic, the smallest amount is sufficient to add a hint of bite, hotting up whatever it singes.

For savoury dishes such as soups and stir-fries add fresh ginger juice by grating the root and squeezing out the liquid in the palm of the hand. The fresh root or dried powder can be used in cakes and desserts, depending on recipe requirements.

Remedial actions of ginger include the treatment of morning and motion sickness, nausea, intestinal gas, indigestion, colds, impaired circulation and aches and pains. Externally, the juice can be applied to cold sores.

To prepare an exhilarating winter tea, grate 25g/1oz of fresh ginger root and simmer in 575ml/1 pint (UK)/1½C (US) of boiling water for 10 minutes. Strain and sip.
Note: ½ heaped tsp of dried ground ginger is equal to 2 heaped tsp of fresh.

### Unusual roots

### Burdock

Although we don't often find burdock dished up, the long, slender root can be steamed and eaten as other roots are. As for its medicinal properties, burdock is a powerful blood purifier and a gentle diuretic and improves skin quality by clearing away blemishes and spots.

## Mooli

Mooli, or daikon as it's otherwise known, is a long white radish, often found in Chinese greengrocers'. It can be grated with carrots and relished as salad or served as a side dish where it aids fat digestion. Mooli also enhances liver detoxification and breaks up catarrh.

## Kuzu

Kuzu is taken from the root of a Japanese vine and in many ways matches the culinary thickening antics of arrowroot. But whilst arrowroot finishes there, kuzu is valued as a kitchen medicine and has long been treated as a panacea in homes of the Orient.

Because kuzu is highly alkaline-forming, it helps neutralize over-acidic conditions and can replace aspirin in the first-aid chest. It also has the knack (like slippery elm) of soothing irritated mucus linings, coming to the rescue of stomach upsets and diarrhoea.

Kuzu root can be found packaged as powdery white irregular lumps. It dissolves easily in cold water, whereupon it can be taken as an antidote, or mixed into soups and sauces to provide a thicker consistency (see page 160).

## Lotus root

This sweet-tasting vegetable can be purchased fresh or dried. As a remedy for respiratory conditions, the dried slices (which can be bought from health-food stores) can be simmered in boiling water, strained and drunk several times a day.

## Dried fruit

Dried fruits allow us the opportunity of having a little sweetness throughout the cold. They make satisfying snacks for adults and children alike, providing us with instant energy, and can be used to sweeten cakes and cookies with their rich fructose content.

Drying is one of the oldest methods of preserving fresh foods, and leaving fruit out in the sun to dry naturally is superior to freezing it, canning it and other more synthetic dehydrating schemes.

Unlike the fresh, dried fruits do not contain large amounts of vitamin C (this water-soluble vitamin is lost in the drying process), but carbohydrate, fibre and mineral content is increased.

With most of the juice eradicated, it's very easy to eat too much dried fruit. For instance, a handful of dried apricots doesn't look very much, but the same amount in fresh form would fill a large bowl. To prevent chewing more than one can handle, it's probably wise to plump them up overnight by soaking them in water and/or stewing them in fruit juice.

Steer clear of fruits coated with inorganic mineral oil, as this interferes with mineral absorption from other foods. Also avoid fruits that are laced with sulphur dioxide, a gas that is sprayed on to prevent them from losing their nice bright colour. Sulphur dioxide destroys vitamin $B_1$ and may produce allergic reactions in sensitive people. It's far better to choose the unsulphured variety, that although doesn't look as appealing tastes just as good.

### Dried fruit

- Apricots are particularly high in the antioxidant beta-carotene.
- Dates (which contain sucrose as their predominant sugar) can be simmered in water until a sweet paste is formed, and used instead of refined, granulated products.
- Figs, unbeknown to many of us, are an excellent source of calcium.
- Prunes and figs help tone up the intestinal tract.
- Dried blueberries facilitate the control of diarrhoea.

*Figure 18, The rich mineral content of dried fruit*

| Dried fruit (per 100g/4oz) | Calcium mg | Magnesium mg | Potassium mg | Sodium mg | Iron mg |
|---|---|---|---|---|---|
| Apples | 31 | 22 | 69 | 5 | 1.6 |
| Apricots | 67 | 62 | 979 | 26 | 5.5 |
| Currants (small seedless grapes) | 87.8 | 37.1 | 747 | 9.1 | 2.5 |
| Dates | 68 | 59 | 750 | 5 | 1.6 |
| Figs | 280 | 92 | 1,010 | 87 | 4.2 |
| Pears | 35 | 31 | 573 | 7 | 1.3 |
| Prunes (plums) | 51 | 59 | 694 | 8 | 1.9 |
| Raisins (grapes) | 54.4 | 35.3 | 673 | 15.6 | 2.1 |
| Sultanas (white seedless grapes) | 52 | 35 | 860 | 53 | 1.8 |
| Average daily needs | 1,500 | 1,000 | 900 | 150 | 15–20 |

# WINTER COOKING TECHNIQUES

In contrast to summer's raw food splendour, winter calls for a mainly cooked regime to keep the inner fire alive.

Steaming, boiling and sautéing can all be applied here, but food that is cooked slowly, over a low heat, will gather a more concentrated vibration, very much in tune with this time of year. Such prolonged methods include baking, roasting, braising and soup making.

### Baking

When we talk of baking, it's understood that food is softened in the oven by way of dry heat. This reduces the moisture content of food, so care should be taken not to let meals dry out. Baking potatoes in their skins, I find, is in winter the most nourishing way to eat them, and with a suitable filling they make a simple, wholesome meal. Baking home-made bread, scones, pasties and sugar-free cakes is also a fitting winter pastime, permeating the kitchen with scrumptious aromas and a radiating cheer.

Before cooking with this technique, first preheat the oven at the recommended temperature for five minutes. Then position the food in the middle shelf until cooked. If browning is required, sit it on the top shelf for a final few minutes.

## Roasting

Roasting, like baking, is also accomplished in the oven, the difference being that the food is glazed with a fine coat of oil. Most winter vegetables can be prepared in this way, delivering a crispness to the outside, whilst revealing a soft, sweet flesh.

Nuts, seeds and flaked cereals can also be lightly roasted, but to avoid them getting burnt it's better to use a thick-bottomed skillet on top of the stove.

## Braising

To braise food, the prepared ingredients need to be placed in a casserole dish half filled with a liquid stock. The dish should then be covered and left to simmer in the oven until the food is soft. Cold-weather hot-pots, casseroles and stews taste extremely desirable cooked by this technique and are definitely worth the long wait.

## Under pressure

Cooking edibles under pressure, with the aid of an appropriate gadget, is an efficient way of softening condensed foods which would otherwise take several hours on the boil. Large legumes are one such item. Cereals and vegetables can also be cooked with this method.

For those of us who go around with our heads in the clouds, or have an over-active imagination, a daily dose of pressure-cooked grain is a sure way of helping to fix our feet firmly back on the ground. This is due to the contractive ('yang') influence, caused by the administration of compression.

## Sensational soups

We can't really cover the mastery of winter cooking without considering the joys of a crusty bread roll and a steaming bowl of soup. Soup-making is the art of combining several foods in a liquid medium, which can be adapted to different times of the year. Whilst summer soups are light, spring soups full of greens and autumn soups dense and vivid, winter soups should be thick and nurturing.

Here are some tools to play around with, to come up with some seasonal soups: vegetables, grains, beans, lentils, split peas, pasta, tofu and seitan.

Legumes should be soaked overnight to shorten the simmering process and vegetables shouldn't be added until the pulses are completely soft. As for grains and pastas, it must be taken into account that extra water will be required, to allow for the expansion of these dried ingredients. Sometimes they can be cooked in a separate saucepan and added to the soup.

*Flavour enhancers* include onions, garlic, celery, celery seeds, spices, herbs, miso, vegetable stock or bouillon, seaweed, tamari and yeast extract. Sauté aromatic vegetables to bring out their flavours. Choose a low or no-salt stock or bouillon. Miso, tamari and fresh herbs are best incorporated when the soup is almost ready, so as not to destroy their piquancy and profit. Adding the right touch of herbs and/or spices can reduce the need for salt.

*Thickeners* include puréed vegetables (potatoes, squash, carrots, parsnips), kuzu root, rolled oats, quinoa, pasta, soya milk, oat milk, nut milk, ground nuts, red split lentils, potato flour and tomato purée. To use kuzu root as a thickener, dissolve 1 heaped tbsp in 4 tbsp (UK)/1⅓C (US) of cold water and add it to an already made soup. Keep it on the heat for a few minutes, until it begins to thicken.

Dairy-free cream soups can be prepared by whizzing the bulk of the soup in a blender, then placing it back into the saucepan and slowly mixing in soya, oat or cashew-nut milk. Give it a heat through and serve.

Small grains, noodles and red lentils also work as thickeners by absorbing excess fluid. Always ensure they are properly cooked.

To concoct a home-made stock, simmer strong-tasting vegetables such as garlic, onion, celery and red pepper, together with seasonal herbs, in water for 45 minutes. Then strain off the solids and use the liquid as stock.

*Seven steps to successful soups*

1 Sauté garlic, chopped onions, leeks, shallots or any other desired pungent plant, in a little oil (1 tbsp (UK)/1½ tbsp (US) maximum) to magnify their zest.
2 Add water and vegetable stock or bouillon and bring to boil.
3 Add the main soup ingredients, allow the liquid to bubble and then, covering with the saucepan lid, leave to simmer.
4 Mix in the required spices.
5 Mix in the required dried herbs.
6 Stir in thickeners if necessary, or if appropriate liquidize the soup in a blender.
7 Add fresh herbs and season.

# FOOD ENERGETICS

When we eat a particular food, it's not just the nutrients that we absorb but the whole energetic value as well. By this, I'm not referring to the Western connotation of fuel or calories, but to the more subtle dietary language of the East.

## Temperature control

Every food, unless categorized as neutral, has the ability to either warm us up or cool us down. For example, fresh fruit or a leafy salad is capable of reducing heat in the body, thus producing a cooling effect. This is caused by the flow of energy within being directed inward and down, fanning the extremities and upper body parts. On the other hand, buckwheat grouts or lentils counteract coldness in the body, by pushing the energy flow upwards and out, and raising the internal thermostat.

However, not everything is this straightforward. Hot spices such as chilli or cayenne, which would generally be perceived as eliciting heat, swing in the opposite direction, quickly cooling us down. This is because when we first eat a spicy meal, the initial

*Figure 19, Some everyday foods and their warming or cooling potential*

| Warming foods | Neutral | Cooling foods |
|---|---|---|
| meat* | brown rice | raw vegetables |
| poultry* | | fresh fruit |
| fish* | | sprouts |
| eggs | | soya beans |
| butter | | mung beans |
| nuts | | tofu |
| seeds | | tempeh |
| lentils | | seaweed |
| beans (most) | | wheat |
| buckwheat | | millet |
| oats | | milk* |
| spelt | | yoghurt |
| quinoa | | tofu |
| corn | | soya milk |
| rye | | chilli |
| dried fruit | | cayenne |
| onion | | herbs |
| garlic | | salt |
| ginger | | sugar* |
| cinnamon | | |
| cloves | | |
| black pepper | | |

*These foods are not recommended.*

Eating too many warming foods, especially animal produce, or not enough cooling ones, may cause a heat condition in the body, leading to symptoms of high blood pressure, inflammatory conditions, skin eruptions, constipation etc.

Eating too many cooling foods, especially excessive quantities of sugar and tropical fruit, or not enough warming foods may over-cool the body, producing symptoms of low blood sugar, diabetes, anorexia, poor circulation etc.

response is so warming that the body starts to perspire, causing heat loss. On this basis, strong spices are best suited to hot climates, where they normally grow.

Now if we take this temperature theory one step further we find that by applying natural altering techniques to a food's basic structure (such as sprouting or cooking), we can change the energetic value of the food.

To illustrate this: if we take adzuki beans, which are potentially warming, we can sprout them so that a cooling food is produced. Again, we can apply heat to tofu or tempeh, preventing its cooling outcome. This manipulatory strategy enables us to convert the quality of certain foods to suit our personal needs.

In the winter we need to eat more warming foods, and in the summer more cooling ones. Ultimately, balance is always the bottom line.

To increase the warming potential of food, use the following heat-producing techniques: cooking; sun-drying; grinding/pounding; chewing. To increase the cooling potential of food, use the following cooling-down techniques: refrigerating; sprouting; juicing.

## WINTER REVIEW

1 Spend more evenings at home and take sufficient rest.
2 Boost the immune system by natural means.
3 Eat lots of cooked, hearty vegetables and grains.
4 Become a soup addict.
5 Drink plenty of therapeutic, herbal teas.
6 Dress up warm and enjoy winter weekend strolls.
7 Learn the art of yoga or t'ai chi.

To conclude our visit to winter, here's a shopping guide to the fresh produce in season. It also includes a variety of dried whole-foods, which although aren't distinct to winter are essential store-cupboard provisions.

*Figure 20, Fresh foods in winter*

| Nuts | Grains | Seeds |
| --- | --- | --- |
| almonds | amaranth | hemp |
| Brazils | barley | linseed |
| cashews | bulgar wheat | pumpkin |
| chestnuts | buckwheat | sesame |
| hazelnuts | maize | sunflower |
| macadamias | millet | |
| peanuts | oats | |
| pecans | quinoa | |
| pine kernels | rice | |
| pistachios | wheat | |
| walnuts | wild rice | |

| Vegetables | Fruit | Herbs | Beans/Pulses |
| --- | --- | --- | --- |
| beetroot | apples | bay leaf | adzuki |
| broccoli | cranberries | marjoram | black turtle |
| Brussels sprouts | pears | rosemary | black-eyed |
| cabbage | rhubarb | sage | borlotti |
| carrots | dried fruit | tarragon | broad |
| celeriac | | thyme | cannellini |
| chicory | | | chickpeas |
| Chinese leaves | | | field |
| cress | | | flageolet |
| garlic | | | haricot |
| globe artichokes | | | mung |
| Jerusalem | | | pinto |
|    artichokes | | | red kidney |
| kale | | | soya |
| kohlrabi | | | lentils |
| leeks | | | split peas |
| mushrooms | | | |
| onions | | | |
| parsnips | | | |
| potatoes | | | |
| radishes | | | |
| swedes or | | | |
|    rutabagas | | | |
| turnips | | | |
| watercress | | | |
| winter squash | | | |

# RECIPES FOR WINTER

### Roast Root Salad
*Serves 6*

INGREDIENTS
900g/2lb parsnips, peeled and trimmed
450g/1lb carrots, peeled and trimmed
4tbsp (UK)/⅓C (US) olive or sesame oil plus a little for oiling
sea salt and black pepper
400g/14oz cooked beetroot, peeled and chopped
Half an onion, peeled and finely chopped
2 heaped tbsp chopped fresh seasonal herbs

Cut the parsnips and carrots into thick chips, place them in an oiled baking dish, brush them with the oil and season with sea salt and pepper. Add a few tablespoons of water to the base to prevent the vegetables from drying out and roast in a preheated oven at 200°C/400°F/Gas 6 for 45 minutes. To ensure they all get crisp, gently turn them halfway through the cooking time. Once cooked, remove from the oven and place in a bowl.

Add the beetroot, onion and herbs to the baked vegetables, mix and serve.

### Garlic, Mushroom and Fennel Salad
*Serves 8*

200g/7oz fancy seasonal lettuce, coarsely shredded
50g/2oz watercress
450g/1lb button mushrooms
8 cloves of garlic, peeled and crushed
6tbsp (UK)/⅔C (US) olive oil
450g/1lb fennel root, halved and finely sliced
sea salt and black pepper

Lay the lettuce in a large salad bowl, and place the watercress on top. In a frying pan, sauté mushrooms and garlic for a few minutes in half the oil until the mushrooms are cooked. Remove them from the pan and put to one side.

In the same pan, sauté the fennel in the remaining oil for about 8–10 minutes, stirring occasionally.

Once cooked, pour the fennel over the watercress, followed by the mushrooms and garlic, season with salt and pepper and serve.

### Roast Potatoes With Triple Bean Topping
*Serves 6*

INGREDIENTS
1.35kg/3lb potatoes, peeled and chopped into large chunks
4tbsp (UK)/⅓C (US) olive oil and a little for oiling
200g/7oz chickpeas, soaked overnight
2 strips of kombu, rehydrated
5 cloves of garlic, peeled and crushed
2tbsp (UK)/3tbsp (US) tahini
sea salt and black pepper
200g/7oz haricot beans, soaked overnight
1 onion, peeled and chopped
100g/4oz carrot, peeled and chopped
75g/3oz celery, chopped
1 heaped tsp paprika
300ml/½pint (UK)/1¼C (US) tomato or mixed vegetable juice
3 dried bay leaves
1 heaped tsp tomato purée
50g/2 oz firm soya cheese

As this dish is made in three layers, separate instructions for each layer are given.

*Potato Layer*

Place the potatoes in an oiled casserole dish, brush with half the olive oil and roast in a preheated oven for 50 minutes at 190°C/375°F/Gas 5. Then set to one side.

## Chickpea layer

Drain the chickpeas, place them in a saucepan of boiling water with half the rehydrated kombu and simmer for two hours or until soft. Once cooked, place them in a bowl with 3 cloves of the garlic and the tahini, sea salt and black pepper and mash with a potato masher. If consistency is too difficult to work with, add a little warm water. When all ingredients are well combined and reasonably soft, spread the mixture evenly over the potatoes.

## Haricot bean layer

Drain the haricot beans, place them in a saucepan of boiling water with the rest of the rehydrated kombu and simmer for 1 hour 30 minutes or until soft. Strain and set aside.

## To assemble

In another saucepan, sauté the onion, carrot, celery, remaining garlic and paprika in the remaining olive oil for 5 minutes. Stir frequently. Then add the tomato or mixed vegetable juice, bay leaves and cooked haricot beans, bring to the boil and simmer for 20 minutes. Add the tomato purée and cook for a further 5 minutes. Season with salt and pepper and pour the bean mixture over the potatoes and chickpea mix. Grate the soya cheese, sprinkle on top and bake in a preheated oven at 190°C/375°F/Gas 5 for 20 minutes. Remove the bay leaves before serving.

## Pumpkin and Chestnut Hot-Pot
*Serves 6*

INGREDIENTS
150g/5oz dried chestnuts, soaked overnight
100g/4oz swede or rutabaga, peeled and chopped
200g/7oz carrots, peeled and chopped
2 cloves of garlic, peeled and crushed
200g/7oz parsnip, peeled and chopped
100g/4oz celery, chopped
450g/1lb potatoes, peeled and chopped
2tbsp (UK)/3tbsp (US) olive oil
100ml/4fl oz (UK)/½C (US) water
½tsp (UK)/½tsp (US) vegetable bouillon
1tsp (UK)/1tsp (US) yeast extract
1 sprig of fresh rosemary
575ml/1 pint (UK)/2½C (US) pumpkin purée
3 heaped tbsp chopped fresh parsley
½ heaped tsp dried thyme

Drain and rinse the chestnuts, place them in a saucepan of boiling water and simmer for 50 minutes until soft. Drain and set aside.

In another saucepan sauté the swede or rutabaga, carrots, garlic, parsnip, celery and potato in the olive oil for 10 minutes, stirring frequently. Add the water, vegetable bouillon, yeast extract and rosemary and simmer on a low heat for 20–25 minutes. Add the pumpkin purée, parsley, thyme and cooked chestnuts and continue to heat for a further five minutes. Serve.

*Note: to save time, pumpkin purée can be purchased already prepared, from most good health-food stores.*

**Red Lentil Lasagne**
*Serves 6–8*

*This delicious vegan lasagne can be adapted to suit those following a gluten-free diet by opting for bread and lasagne sheets made from non-gluten grains.*

225g/8oz onion, peeled and chopped
300g/11oz carrots, peeled and chopped
2 cloves of garlic, peeled and crushed
3 tbsp (UK)/¼C (US) olive oil
750ml/27fl oz (UK)/3½C (US) tomato or mixed vegetable juice
250g/9oz red split lentils[2]
1 sprig of fresh rosemary
½tsp (UK)/½tsp (US) vegetable bouillon
400ml/14fl oz (UK)/1¾C (US) water
6 heaped tbsp chopped fresh flat-leaf parsley
1½ heaped tsp dried oregano
2tsp (UK)/2tsp (US) tamari
200g/7oz kale, chopped
550g/1¼lb plain firm tofu
1 heaped tsp paprika powder
1 heaped tbsp freeze-dried coriander leaf
sea salt
200g/7oz pre-cooked spinach lasagne, fresh or dried
200g/7oz breadcrumbs of choice
1 heaped tsp mustard powder
black pepper
200g/7oz vegetarian goat's Cheddar or firm soya cheese, grated

In a saucepan, sauté the onion, carrots and garlic in the olive oil. When the onions are transparent add the tomato or mixed vegetable juice, lentils, rosemary and vegetable bouillon, bring to the boil and simmer for 10 minutes then add water and continue to cook for a further 20 minutes. Towards the end of the cooking time, add the parsley, oregano and tamari. In another saucepan steam the kale for 8–10 minutes and mix into the lentil sauce.

Mash the tofu with a potato masher, mix in the paprika, coriander and sea salt and set aside.

In a 30mm/12in × 23mm/9in × 6mm/2½in lasagne dish spread a

third of the lentil sauce evenly in the bottom and cover with half of the mashed tofu. Place a layer of spinach lasagne on top. Repeat the layers a second time. Place the remaining lentil sauce on top of lasagne. Mix the breadcrumbs with the mustard powder and black pepper and sprinkle over the top. Add the grated cheese and bake in a preheated oven at 190°C/375°F/Gas 5 for 25–30 minutes.

### Kasha with Nuts and Raisins
*Serves* 6

INGREDIENTS
100g/4oz roasted buckwheat groats
One 325g/12oz can of sweetcorn kernels, drained
half an onion, peeled and very finely chopped
75g/3oz celery, chopped
75g/3oz pecan nuts or nuts of choice
50g/2oz raisins
1 clove of garlic, peeled and crushed
Dressing
2tbsp (UK)/3tbsp (US) tahini
1tsp UK/2tsp (US) tamari
sea salt and black pepper
2tbsp water

Simmer the buckwheat groats in twice the volume of boiling water for 10 minutes. Once soft, place in a bowl, add the sweetcorn, onion, celery, nuts, raisins and garlic and mix.

Combine the dressing ingredients and stir into the buckwheat.

## Vegetable Nori Tempura
*Serves 6–8*

*This is one of my very rare deep-fried recipes. Use the vegetables below or any other vegetables in season.*

sea salt
100g/4oz spelt flour, sieved
50g/2oz arrowroot flour
1 heaped tsp mustard flour
2 heaped tbsp nori flakes
300ml/½ pint (UK)/1¼C (US) water
300ml/½ pint (UK)/1¼C (US) sesame oil (or enough for deep frying)
250g/9oz parsnips, peeled and cut into chips
250g/9oz sweet potatoes, peeled and cut into chips
200g/7oz carrots, peeled and cut into chips
250g/9oz broccoli, cut into small florets

Combine the sea salt, spelt flour, arrowroot flour and mustard flour in a bowl, add the nori flakes and the water and mix into a batter. Heat the oil in a small saucepan or deep-frying pan, taking care that the oil doesn't smoke.

When the oil is hot enough dip the chipped vegetables into the batter and one by one, drop them into the oil. Leave to fry for a few minutes until light golden brown. Drain off excess oil on kitchen paper and serve immediately.

## Swede-Topped Adzuki Casserole
*Serves* 6

INGREDIENTS
200g/7oz adzuki beans, soaked overnight
1 piece of kombu, rehydrated
1 onion, peeled and chopped
1tbsp (UK)/1½tbsp (US) olive oil
1 clove of garlic, peeled and crushed
150g/5oz Brussels sprouts, outer leaves removed, and halved
1 heaped tbsp paprika
200ml/7fl oz (UK)/scant 1C (US) water
2tsp (UK)/2tsp (US) vegetable bouillon
One 400g/14oz tin of artichoke hearts, drained and halved
1 heaped tbsp dried oregano
2tsp (UK)/2tsp (US) barley miso
350g/12oz swede or rutabaga, peeled and chopped
350g/12oz potato, peeled and chopped
1 heaped tsp unhydrogenated margarine
sea salt and black pepper

Drain the beans, place them in a saucepan of water with the strip of kombu, bring to the boil and simmer for one hour, until soft. Set aside.

In another saucepan, sauté the onions in the olive oil until they are transparent. Add the garlic, Brussels sprouts and paprika and stir. Pour in the water and vegetable bouillon and simmer for 10 minutes. Mix in the artichoke hearts, adzuki beans, oregano and miso and continue to simmer for a further few minutes until ingredients are evenly distributed. Pour into a casserole dish and leave to one side.

Steam the swede or rutabaga and potatoes for 20 minutes until soft. Add margarine and seasoning and mash until smooth. Spread over the bean and vegetable mixture and bake in a preheated oven at 190°C/375°F/Gas 5 for 30 minutes.

**Lentil and Brazil Nut Roast**
*Serves 6–8*

INGREDIENTS
100g/4oz black turtle beans, soaked overnight
1 strip of kombu, rehydrated
200g/7oz green lentils, soaked overnight
1 onion, peeled and chopped
100g/4oz celery, finely chopped
200g/7oz carrots, peeled and grated
2tbsp (UK)/3tbsp (US) olive oil
2tsp(UK)/2tsp (US) tamari
½tsp (UK)/½tsp (US) yeast extract
2 heaped tsp dried sage
1 heaped tsp dried thyme
4 heaped tbsp chopped fresh parsley
1tbsp (UK)/1½tbsp (US) tomato purée
1 heaped tbsp arrowroot flour

Drain and rinse black turtle beans and simmer in boiling water with the kombu for 1 hour. Remove soak water from lentils and simmer in boiling water for 25 minutes. When both are soft, drain and mash them together in a large basin.

Sauté the onion, celery and carrot in the olive oil for 5 minutes, add the tamari and yeast extract and simmer for a few minutes until the vegetables are soft. Pour into the bean and lentil basin, add all remaining ingredients and mix so that everything is well blended. This can be done in a food mixer if available.

Place into an oiled 900g/2lb loaf tin, cover with foil and bake in a preheated oven at 180°C/350°F/Gas 4 for 2 hours. To crisp up the top, the foil can be removed in the final 10 minutes of cooking time.

**Barley Miso Soup**
*Serves* 6

INGREDIENTS
200g/7oz onions, peeled and chopped
200g/7oz carrots, peeled and cut into small sticks
1 heaped tbsp paprika
2tbsp (UK)/3tbsp (US) sesame oil
1.5 litres/2½ pints (UK)/6¼C (US) water
100g/4oz pot barley, soaked overnight and drained
3 strips of wakame, chopped and rehydrated
100g/4oz greens (whatever is in season)
2–3tbsp (UK)/3tbsp–¼C (US) barley miso

In a large saucepan sauté the onions, carrots and paprika in the oil for a few minutes until the onions are transparent. Stir frequently to prevent burning. Add the water, barley, wakame and greens, bring to the boil and simmer on a very low flame for an hour. If more water is needed, add as required. Stir in the barley miso, heat through and serve.

**Spicy Winter Vegetable Soup**
*Serves* 6

*This is wonderful eaten with warm bread.*

INGREDIENTS
1 medium kabocha squash, or other variety if unavailable
2 tbsp (UK)/3tbsp (US) olive or sesame oil
100g/4oz leek, trimmed and cut into thin strips
1 clove of garlic, peeled and crushed
1–2 heaped tbsp paprika powder
1 heaped tbsp mustard seeds
200g/7oz sweet potato, peeled and chopped
1 litre/1¾ pints (UK)/4½C (US) water
200g/7oz swede or rutabaga, peeled and chopped
1 strip of kombu, hydrated
¼ heaped tsp mild chilli powder
black pepper

Cut the squash in half horizontally, remove and discard the seeds, brush the flesh with a little of the oil and bake face down in a preheated oven 205°C/400°F/Gas 6 for 40–50 minutes, until soft. Set aside.

In a large saucepan, sauté the leeks in the remaining oil for 5 minutes. Add the garlic, paprika, mustard seeds and sweet potato and continue to fry for a further few minutes, stirring frequently. Then add the water, swede or rutabaga, the flesh from the baked squash, kombu and chilli powder and simmer for 35–40 minutes.

Finally, with a potato masher, mash down the vegetables, leaving some slightly chunky, simmer for a further 5 minutes, season with pepper and serve.

## Apple, Sesame and Ginger Crumble
*Serves 6*

900g/2lb apples, cored and chopped into small pieces
200ml/7fl oz (UK)/scant 1C (US) apple juice
2tbsp (UK)/3tbsp (US) maple syrup
50g/2oz jumbo oats
50g/2oz rolled oats
50g/2oz oatbran
4 heaped tbsp sesame seeds
1 heaped tsp ginger powder
¼ heaped tsp nutmeg
50g/2oz unhydrogenated sunflower margarine

Simmer the apples in the juice for 15 minutes or until the juice is absorbed, adding the maple syrup towards the end of the cooking time. Once soft, place the apple mixture in a baking dish.

In a saucepan combine the jumbo oats, rolled oats, oatbran and sesame seeds and toast over a small flame, stirring all the time. Add the ginger and nutmeg and work in the margarine until the ingredients are well combined. Spread the crumble mixture on top of the apples and bake in a preheated oven at 190°C/375°F/Gas 5 for 25 minutes.

## Dried Fruit Compôte with Almond Whip
*Serves 6*

INGREDIENTS
450g/1lb dried mixed fruit, including apples, apricots, figs,
peaches, pears and prunes, soaked overnight in apple juice
275g/10oz plain firm tofu
5tbsp (UK)/½C (US) maize or brown rice syrup
50g/2oz almonds
1tsp (UK)/1tsp (US) natural vanilla essence
⅛tsp (UK)/⅛tsp (US) natural almond essence
75ml/3fl oz (UK)/⅓C (US) sunflower oil

Drain the dried fruit reserving 100ml/4fl oz (UK)/½C (US) of the juice,
and set the fruit aside. In a blender, whizz half of the tofu with the
reserved juice. Add the rice malt, almonds, natural essences, remaining
tofu and oil and blend until very thick and smooth. Chill and serve on
top of the dried fruit.

# A Final Word

'The Human Seasons'

*Four Seasons fill the measure of the year;*
*There are four seasons in the mind of man:*
*He has his lusty Spring, when fancy clear*
*Takes in all beauty with an easy span;*
*He has his Summer, when luxuriously*
*Spring's honied cud of youthful thought he loves*
*To ruminate, and by dreaming high*
*Is nearest unto heaven: quiet coves*
*His soul has in its Autumn, when his wings*
*He furleth close; contented so to look*
*On mists in idleness – to let fair things*
*Pass by unheeded as a threshold brook*
*He has his Winter too of pale misfeature,*
*Or else he would forgo his mortal nature.*

JOHN KEATS

Well, that's it – our journey is over. I hope you've enjoyed the trip through the seasons as much as I enjoyed writing about it.

Just a quick word before closing. Follow the seasonal guidelines as best you can – but avoid becoming overly rigid. If the occasional out-of-season item is required, then let it pass – it won't be the end of the world. Or if you have a passion for a pineapple or papaya and you live in a temperate zone, then so be it – just don't make it a habit.

Being completely inflexible can sometimes cause as much illness as not caring at all. The main aim is to stick to the basics of wholefoods, and enjoy what you eat.

Season's Greetings and Happy Eatings

Paula Bartimeus

# Notes

## Chapter 1

1 The acid/alkaline potential of a food is not a reflection of its acid/alkaline content, but rather the ash it leaves after being burnt.
2 Due to the presence of acid-forming substances in spinach, chard, kale and beet greens, eaten regularly in large amounts these vegetables may eventually cause an acid response.
3 The oils in the alkaline and slightly acid categories apply only to those that are completely unrefined and in their raw state.
4 A paper issued by Natural Justice Limited reviews the evidence which correlates nutritional status with antisocial and criminal tendencies. Further information is available from Natural Justice Limited, 1 Trinity Hall, The Gill, Ulverston, Cumbria, LA12 7BJ.

## Chapter 2

1 Horticulturally buckwheat, quinoa and amaranth are not true grains, but can be prepared and used in the same way as other cereals.
2 Botanically, rhubarb is actually a vegetable, but because of the way it is used, it's most often portrayed as a fruit.
3 Aflatoxin may also affect almonds, Brazil nuts, pecans, pistachios and walnuts, although organically raised specimens are less likely to harbour this poison.

## Chapter 3

1 These findings also apply to other refined items such as polished grains and white flour products.

2 When using herbal teas as curatives, they should be drunk at least three times a day.

## Chapter 4

1 Moreover, the warming attributes of winter crops can be amplified by cooking.

## Chapter 5

1 I have adapted certain Chinese concepts – such as there being five seasons – to fit in with the predominantly Western perspective and flow of this book.

## Chapter 6

1 The official dates laid down for each season are in accord with Greenwich Mean Time (GMT) and relates to Northern-hemisphere countries. Times may vary slightly by several hours, depending on year and location. For countries that lie in the Southern half of the planet, the seasons and dates are reversed: eg 20 March signifies spring in the North and autumn in the South.
2 Seeds used for sprouting must be whole. Those that are refined, split or rolled will not germinate.
3 The bouillon that I use is a reduced salt, dried variety.

## Chapter 7

1 Exceptions being those varieties of apples and pear cultivars which have been specially bred for picking and later ripening; early-ripening apples are usually gathered before they are fully ripe or the fruits may become mealy. A variety such as, for example, Bramley's Seedling may be used November to March (UK winter to spring). Medlars are also fruit which cannot be eaten until bletted.
2 Fruits such as dates and grapes may not grow naturally in places such as Britain but do grow in many other temperate countries – which is why I have included them in this list.

3 Tofu which has already been marinated (usually in ginger and soya sauce) can be purchased from most health food stores.

## Chapter 8

1 Although the majority of sea vegetables are imported from small Japanese suppliers, other sources originate from the Northern Pacific in both Asia and America and the Northern Atlantic, in both America and Europe.
2 Another type of kombu, otherwise tagged as kelp, is found in the Atlantic and most often sold as a nutritional supplement in the form of a powder or tablets.
3 Soba is long, flat strips of pasta.

## Chapter 9

1 This means deep- *and* shallow-fried food. When the recipes in this book refer to sautéing, it's in the minimum amount of oil (not enough for shallow-frying) for the minimum amount of time.
2 Red split lentils are small and cook quickly. They don't need to be pre-cooked or soaked beforehand.

# Further Reading

Alexander, Jane, *The Natural Year*, Bantam Books, 1997

Colbin, Annemarie, *Food And Healing*, Ballantine Books, New York, 1986

Cousens, Gabriel, *Conscious Eating*, Essene Vision Books, Patagonia, Arizona, 1992

Erasmus, Udo, *Fats That Heal Fats That Kill*, Alive Books, Burnaby, Canada, 1986

Grant, Doris and Jean Joice, *Food Combining For Health*, Thorsons, London, 1984

Hanssen, Maurice, *The Complete Raw Juice Therapy*, Thorsons, London, 1989

Haas, Elson M, MD, *Staying Healthy With The Seasons*, Celestial Arts, Berkeley, California, 1981

Jensen, Dr Bernard, *Foods That Heal*, Avery Publishing, New York, 1988

Klaper, Michael, MD, *Vegan Nutrition: Pure And Simple*, Gentle World, Inc, Maui, 1995

Le Tissier, Jackie, *Food Combining For Vegetarians*, Thorsons, London, 1992

Moore Lappe, Francis, *Diet For A Small Planet*, Ballantine Books, New York, 1971

Murray, Michael T, *The Healing Power Of Foods*, Prima Publishing, Rocklin, California, 1993

Michell, Keith, *The Practically Macrobiotic Cookbook*, Thorsons, London, 1987

Tierra, Michael, *The Way Of Herbs*, Pocket Books, New York, 1980

Turner, Kristina, *The Self Healing Cookbook*, Earthtones Press, Vashon Island, 1987

# Bibliography

## BOOKS

Adolphus, Margaret, *Garlic, Nature's Remedy*, Nutri-HealthData Ltd, Milton Keynes, 1991

Ballentine, Rudolph MD, *Diet and Nutrition*, The Himalayan International Institute, Pennsylvania, 1978

Batmanghelidj, F. MD, *The Body's Many Cries For Water* Global Health Solutions Inc, Falls Church, Virginia, 1992

Belleme, John and Jan, *Culinary Treasures Of Japan*, Avery Publishing, New York, 1992

Berry, Linda, *A Practical Guide To Colon Health*, Botanica Press, Capitola, 1985

Bradford, Peter and Montse, *Cooking With Sea Vegetables*, Healing Arts Press, Vermont, 1985

Carper, Jean, *Food Your Miracle Medicine*, Simon and Schuster, London, 1993

Chevallier, Andrew, *Herbal Teas*, Amberwood Publishing Ltd, Surrey, 1994

Colbin, Annemarie, *Food And Healing*, Ballantine Books, New York, 1986

Cole, Candia Lea, *Super Smoothies*, Woodbridge Press, Santa Barbara, 1996

Colgan, Dr Michael, *The New Nutrition*, CI Publications, San Diego, 1994

Connelly, Dianne M, *Traditional Acupuncture: The Law Of The Five Elements*, The Centre For Traditional Acupuncture, Maryland, 1979

*Country Life Cookbook*, MMI Press, Harrisville, 1984

Cousens, Gabriel, MD, *Conscious Eating*, Essene Vision Books, Patagonia, Arizona, 1992

Cousens, Gabriel, MD, *Spiritual Nutrition And The Rainbow Diet*, Cassandra Press, San Rafael, California, 1986

Cowmeadow, Oliver, *Introduction to Macrobiotics*, Thorsons, Northamptonshire, 1987

Erasmus, Udo, *Fats That Heal Fats That Kill*, Alive Books, Burnaby, Canada, 1986

Fallon, Sally, *Nourishing Traditions*, Promotion Publishing, San Diego, 1995

Fox, Brian A, and Cameron, Allan G, *Food Science, Nutrition and Health*, Edward Arnold, London, 1961

Goulart, Frances Sheridon, *Super Healing Foods*, Parker Publishing Company, New York, 1995

Gray, Robert, *The Colon Health Handbook*, Emerald Publishing, Nevada, 1980

Hanssen, Maurice, *The Complete Raw Juice Therapy*, Thorsons, London, 1987

Haas, Elson M, MD, *Staying Healthy With The Seasons*, Celestial Arts, Berkeley, California, 1981

*Holford, Patrick,* Living Foods, ION Press, London, 1996

Hunter, Beatrice Trum, *Grain Power*, Keats Publishing Inc, Connecticut, 1994

Jensen, Dr Bernard, *Foods That Heal*, Avery Publishing, New York, 1988

Kenton, Leslie, *Passage To Power*, Vermilion, London, 1995

Klaper, Michael, MD, *Vegan Nutrition: Pure And Simple*, Gentle World Inc, Maui, 1995

Kloss, Jethro, *Back To Eden*, Back To Eden Books, California, 1939

Kordich, Jay, *The Juiceman's Power of Juicing*, Warner Books, New York, 1993

Kushi, Michio, *The Book Of Macro-biotics*, Japan Publications Inc, New York, 1977

Kushi, Aveline, and Esko, Wendy, *The Changing Seasons Macrobiotic Cookbook*, Avery, New Jersey, 1995

Le Tissier, Jackie, *Food Combining For Vegetarians*, Thorsons, London, 1992

Meyerowitz, Steve, *Sprout It!* The Sprout House, Great Barrington, 1983

Moore Lappe, Frances, *Diet For A Small Planet*, Ballantine Books, New York, 1971

Murray, Michael T, *The Healing Power Of Foods*, Prima Publishing, Rocklin, California, 1993

Pickarski, Brother Ron, *Friendly Foods*, Ten Speed Press, Berkeley, California, 1991

Pitchford, Paul, *Healing With Whole Foods*, North Atlantic Books, Berkeley, California, 1993

Ridgeway, Judy, *Sprouting Beans and Seeds*, Century Publishing, London, 1994

Rinzler, Carol Ann, *Herbs, Spices and Condiments*, Henry Holt, New York, 1990

Soloman, Jay, *Vegetarian Soup Cuisine*, Prima Publishing, Rocklin, California, 1996

Stovel, Edith, *Salt-Free Herb Cookery*, Storey, Vermont, 1985

Tierra, Michael, *EastWeat Master Course In Herbology*, Santa Cruz, California, 1981

Tierra, Michael, *The Way Of Herbs*, Pocket Books, New York, 1980

Turner, Kristina, *The Self Healing Cookbook*, Earthtones Press, Vashon Island, 1987

Walker, Dr N W, *The Vegetarian Guide To Diet and Salad*, Norwalk Press, Arizona, 1940

## MAGAZINES, PAPERS AND PUBLICATIONS

Bartimeus, Paula, 'Take Six Seaweeds', *Here's Health*, Dec 1995

Bartimeus, Paula, 'Go With The Grain', *Here's Health*, April 1996

Bartimeus, Paula, 'Bean Power', *Here's Health*, 1996

Blythman, Joanna, 'Local Heroes', *BBC Vegetarian*.

Brown, Linda, 'Kitchen Garden Patch Work', *BBC Vegetarian*.

Buswell, Leonie, *ION Research*, Volume 9 Number 6, Autumn 1996

Connor, Steve, 'Fatal Foods', *Here's Health*, December 1996

Diamond, Sandra, 'Summer Leaves', *Here's Health*, August 1994

Doves Farm, 'Spelt – An Ancient Breadmaking Flour' (pamphlet)

Fresh Fruit and Vegetable Information Bureau, 'Fresh Fruit and Vegetables – Availability In UK etc 'Pumpkins and Squashes', 'Celeriac', 'Fennel', 'Jerusalem Artichokes', 'Asparagus', 'Marrows'

The Herb Society, 'Drying Herbs', Information sheet Number 1

Holford, Patrick, 'Breakthroughs In Nutrition', *Beyond Nutrition*, Issue 1
Holford, Patrick, 'Are Meat And Milk Safe to Eat?' *Optimum Nutrition*, Volume 9 Number 1, Spring 1996
Holford, Patrick, 'Eau No', *Optimum Nutrition*, Volume 3 Number 3, Autumn 1990
Hollis, Liz, 'Chemical Cocktails', *Healthy Eating*, October 1995
Lilly, Ravinder, 'Get Fruity', *Healthy Eating*, October 1995
MacDonald, Heather, 'Don't Be SAD', *Here's Health*, December 1995
'Skin Brushing', Larkhall Green Farm, 702N (pamphlet)
Terrass, Stephen, 'Phytonutrients, A Solgar Reference Manual'
'Toxins in Your Food', *Which?*, August 1994

# Useful Addresses

## BRITAIN

The Institute of Allergy Therapists
Llangwyryfon
Aberystwyth
Dyfed SY23 4EY
Tel: 01974 241376

Clearspring Ltd
19A Acton Park Estate
London W3 7QE
Tel: 0181 749 1781
(sea vegetable importers)

College Of Natural Nutrition
1 Halthaies
Bradninch
Nr Exeter
Devon EX 54LQ
Tel: 01392 881091

Community Health Foundation
188 Old Street
London EC1V 9FR
Tel: 0171 251 4076
(macrobiotic centre)

Fruit and Vegetable Information Bureau
Bury House
126–128 Cromwell Road
London SW7 4ET
Tel: 0171 373 7734

Revital Health
3A The Colonnades
Buckingham Palace Road
London SW1W 9RZ
Tel: 0171 976 6615
(All specialized foods and supplements mentioned in this book can be
purchased from this above address.)

SAD (Seasonal Affective Disorder Helpline)
10 Brunswick Street
Bath BA1 6PQ
Tel: 01225 317429

Soil Association
86 Colston Street
Bristol BS1 5BB
Tel: 0117 929 0661

Vegan Society
7 Battle Road
St Leonards-on-Sea
East Sussex TN37 7AA
Tel: 01424 427393

Vegetarian Society
Parkdale
Dunham
Altrincham
Cheshire WA14 4QG
Tel: 0161 928 0793

# AMERICA

North American Vegetarian Society
PO Box 72
Dolgeville NY 13329

American Vegan Society
56 Dinshah Lane
Malaga NJ 08328

East-West Foundation
PO Box 850
Brookline MA 02147

George Ohsawa Macrobiotic Foundation
1999 Myers Street
Oroville
CA 95966

Maine Coast Sea Vegetables
Shore Road
Franklin
Maine 04634

California Certified Organic Farmers
1115 Mission Street
Santa Cruz
California 95061

The Natural Gourmet Cookery School
48 West 21st Street
Second Floor
New York, NY 10010

# AUSTRALIA

Australian Vegetarian Society
PO Box 65
Paddington
New South Wales 2021

The Vegan Society
PO Box 85
Seaford
Victoria 3198

Australian College of Natural Medicine
362 Water Street
Fortitude Valley QLD 4006

Australian College of Nutritional and Environmental Medicine
13 Hilton Street
Deakin ACT 2600

Hippocrates Health Centre
Elaine Avenue
Parramatta
NSW 2150

# NEW ZEALAND

The New Zealand Vegetarian Society
PO Box 77-034
Auckland 3

# SOUTH AFRICA

The Vegetarian Society of South Africa
PO Box 15091
Lambton 1414

# Index